FOOD WITHOUT FEAR

Identify, Prevent, and Treat Food Allergies, Intolerances, and Sensitivities

Ruchi Gupta, MD, MPH
with Kristin Loberg

Where are you on the food sensitivity spectrum?

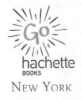

hachette
BOOKS
NEW YORK

*To the fearless individuals and families in my daily work who inspire me,
and to my devout team who turns those inspirations into reality.*

Copyright © 2021 by Ruchi Gupta, MD, MPH

Cover design by Terri Sirma
Cover photographs © Science Photo Library/Getty; Science Photo Library/
Shutterstock; Eggs, soybeans, avocado, shrimp/Shutterstock
Cover copyright © 2021 by Hachette Book Group, Inc.

Hachette Go, an imprint of Hachette Books
Hachette Book Group
1290 Avenue of the Americas
New York, NY 10104
HachetteGo.com
Facebook.com/HachetteGo
Instagram.com/HachetteGo

First Edition: August 2021

Hachette Books is a division of Hachette Book Group, Inc.

The Hachette Go and Hachette Books name and logos are trademarks of Hachette
Book Group, Inc.

The publisher is not responsible for websites (or their content) that are not owned
by the publisher.

Print book interior design by Linda Mark.

Library of Congress Cataloging-in-Publication Data has been applied for.

ISBNs: 978-0-306-84650-2 (hardcover); 978-0-306-84649-6 (ebook)

Printed in the United States of America

LSC-C

Printing 1, 2021

CONTENTS

---------------------------------- PART II ----------------------------------

FINDING FOOD FREEDOM:
IDENTIFY AND EMPOWER; TREAT;
MANAGE AND PREVENT; AND THRIVE

INTRODUCTION

Welcome to Food Freedom

M Y PHONE RANG OFF THE HOOK. IT WAS THE BEGINNING OF 2019 AND mainstream media had just reported that more than 10 percent of adults in the US—over 26 million people—are estimated to have food allergy, and almost twice as many individuals—52 million—believe they have food allergy but may have another food-related condition. Up to 85 million are avoiding certain foods due to food conditions. They use the term *food allergy* very loosely for many conditions that are not considered to be allergies in the medical community. And the words *sensitivity* and *intolerance* further cause confusion.

It was my research that produced these new surprising numbers, and everyone wanted to know *why*—how is this possible? Where's the smoking gun? The other shocker my epidemiological sleuthing found is that nearly half of adults with food allergy developed the condition during adulthood, which went patently against conventional wisdom that said allergies start in childhood. More questions came flooding in: What's going on? How can we suddenly have so many challenges with food when not much has changed in our lifestyles and relationship with food? *Or has it?* What is to blame? Where is the source? And what explains food's unexpected turn on a grown adult (who likely has been eating the now troublesome food for decades)?

Indeed, I had my work cut out for me, alongside the many other curious doctors and researchers around the world. This was my opportunity to change the stereotypes around food allergy and get to the bottom of this growing epidemic. Luckily, these findings have coalesced with remarkable new therapies and technologies in medicine to identify, treat, and manage all kinds of food-related issues. At the same time, we're rapidly learning how best to prevent allergic diseases and their relatives altogether.

Admittedly, unraveling the mysteries of food allergies was not always my passion or mission. Early in my career, my research focused primarily on asthma until I met a family in 2004 with two young children struggling with food allergies. It was an eye-opening and empowering experience for me. At that time, little did I know that as I dove into this largely uncharted territory, my work would so profoundly overlap with my personal life.

One day in the spring of 2006, my son was playing with my daughter, in between munching on a peanut butter and jelly sandwich. He was five and she was one. With his sticky fingers, he must have unknowingly touched her mouth and face. She soon broke out into hives on her face spreading down her neck and body, followed by vomiting. That was my first introduction to food allergies from a caregiver's perspective. It was both shocking and terrifying. That day changed my—and my daughter's—life forever. From that moment on, food allergy management and research became a 24-7 job for me. I live it every day—I see patients with it, I conduct studies on it, I debunk myths about it to the young and old, and I come home to it.

Anyone who has or knows someone with food allergies or a food-related condition sees the world differently. Life suddenly becomes a minefield of potential hazards. You don't know where the next chance encounter with a problematic ingredient will come from, how bad the reaction will be, and whether it will involve (another) trip to the bathroom, pharmacy, or emergency room. Food is everywhere and encompasses so much in our culture—from how we nourish ourselves daily just to survive, to how we celebrate special milestones and holidays throughout the year. We enjoy the company of others over food; plan events, outings, and gatherings around food; and make it a central part of our very being and happiness. Eating is a part of life no one can avoid, so when food becomes something to fear, life takes on a whole new meaning where allaying or ending those fears is tantamount.

Even if a food is not supposed to have a certain allergic ingredient, there's always the risk of cross-contact or accidental exposure—that dollop of chocolate ice cream served from the same scoop used for pistachio and hazelnut ice cream. A kale chip dusted in cashew powder. An expansive buffet table with unsuspecting dishes prepared using sesame oil and seeds. The number of times I have been confused about the potential safety of a food, second-guessed a food label, watched an individual's palpable fear over food, and have been generally worried is, frankly, enough to drive anybody nuts (no pun intended).

I wrote this book amid the Covid-19 pandemic. During this stressful time, we've all had to be extra mindful and careful about what we touch, where we go, with whom we socialize, how far we stand from potential sources of contaminants, how we engage in public settings (especially bars and restaurants), and what air we breathe. When you think about it, such hypervigilance is not that new for people with food allergies. However, unlike during the Covid-19 crisis, people with food allergies may have their condition for life and will continue to live this way long after the pandemic. The food allergy epidemic is exceedingly complex, and the fact that diagnosing the various food-related conditions across the entire spectrum is neither straightforward nor foolproof further muddies the waters.

The spectrum! As my research into food allergies grows, it has become so evident that there is an ever-expanding list of conditions, many with unclear causes, that often get lumped into this terminology *food allergy*, although they may have a different mechanism of action in the body. In this book, we will refer to this myriad of food conditions as "masqueraders"—other conditions that may cause symptoms after eating particular foods but do not include the biological (immune-based) reactions characteristic of food allergy (and are thus categorized differently in medicine).

In the present era of medicine and molecular diagnostics (e.g., DNA sequencing of tumors to look for mutations that match potential drug therapies to control cancer), our ability to accurately and reliably diagnose our patients' suspected food allergies and especially these masqueraders is not great. We don't yet have easy tests that can provide clear, infallible answers and, in turn, treatment plans and cures. Patients and their families frequently express frustration about our inability to conclusively diagnose their food-related problems. Masqueraders are not usually life-threatening, but they can cause uncomfortable symptoms from gas, bloating, nausea, and diarrhea, to rashes, an itchy mouth, nasal congestion, and headaches—much like many food allergies, so it is easy to understand the confusion.

To say this epidemic has many fuzzy boundaries is an understatement. Similar to the field of cancer, there are many different "types" and "subtypes" of food-related conditions, and yet we must address this area of medicine as a collective whole. The epidemic will not end unless we take a broad approach, factor in all the variables, and embrace new ways of thinking. The potential upshots are infinite. You never know how solving one problem in this intricate picture can help solve another problem elsewhere in the grand picture of human health and wellness. In this larger picture, the sum is greater than its parts.

What can help us better understand this epidemic and treat the problem is a revolutionary way to think about it: *as a food reaction spectrum*. On one extreme, we have serious food allergies that incite the immune system in dramatic ways and send people to emergency rooms, unable to swallow or breathe. At the other extreme, we have intolerances (or "sensitivities"—we'll get to these important definitions shortly) to foods that don't necessarily involve the immune system at all yet diminish people's quality of life because their condition prevents them from enjoying certain foods without such symptoms as intestinal distress, low energy, or migraines. Their lives are also disrupted on a daily basis as they shoulder the added weight of making smart food choices to avoid painful physical suffering. And then there's everything in between these two extremes that can be convoluted, overlapping, and confusing.

Adding to this tangled picture are conditions unrelated to food but where symptoms may seem related to food due to their effects on the digestive system. For example, gastrointestinal illnesses, such as ulcerative colitis and Crohn's disease—both of which belong to a group of conditions under inflammatory bowel disease (IBD)—can involve symptoms that closely mimic those of food allergy or intolerances. Specific foods may aggravate these conditions, but they do not cause them and should be treated separately. As we'll see in Chapter 4, conditions as seemingly far afield from food allergy as autoimmune diseases, cardiovascular ailments, and even cancer could share surprising connections in the intricate hidden highways within the body. (Spoiler alert: Your body's inflammatory pathways and immune function are huge driving forces whether we're talking about classic food allergy, a skin condition, or an autoimmune disorder. Aside from the well-established relationship between eczema [atopic dermatitis] and allergies, other skin disorders can share features with food-related issues, particularly intolerances; people who swear that certain foods, such as milk, refined carbs, and sugar, trigger acne, for example, are probably not imagining it. Scientists are still figuring out these connections but no doubt they involve systems and cascades in the body that relate with one another.)

One person can have just a single, somewhat isolated issue with one particular ingredient that's easily avoidable, and someone else can have multiple issues all at once under the same gigantic umbrella—asthma, eczema, hay fever, intolerance to lactose and sulfites, problems with caffeine, pollen-food allergy syndrome (PFAS, a.k.a. oral allergy syndrome [OAS]) to fruits, or allergy to tree nuts, peanuts, sesame, and eggs (raw, not baked). As you can appreciate, it gets complicated, but by formatting the matter around a spectrum, we can put this into clear perspective and offer a range of solutions. It's a groundbreaking approach to thinking about and addressing the epidemic like never before. This book presents a start to understanding this spectrum. It is by no means complete as we are learning more about the conditions, their categorization, and their relationship every day.

My goal is to take the fear out of living with food-related challenges. Indeed, the fear factor can be debilitating—fear of dining out, fear of going to a dinner party, fear of managing reactions at work, fear of sharing food with anyone else, fear of travel and vacationing, fear of sending a kid to a sleepover, to camp, to a theme park, to a sports game in a large stadium, or to grandma's house, and fear of eating in general. For nearly two decades now, I've made it my main priority to improve the lives of children, adults, and families living with food allergy and other food-related conditions, and to reduce the fear and confusion that comes along with them.

Back when I first began my work in this field, thanks to my introduction to those first families with food allergies, I quickly realized how much we didn't know about these conditions, and how much research was still needed. It was one of those relatively new, poorly understood, and rapidly increasing areas in medicine in need of greater knowledge and clarity using the power of modern, twenty-first-century research capabilities. I was seeing more and more patients with food allergy, and I had very few resources and information available to share with them as they navigated their difficult new lifestyle faced with the unknown. I was determined to change that. I had the privilege of listening to these patients' stories firsthand, and these conversations helped me understand where the big holes in research were and where we needed to go next.

The questions began swirling in my head: How many people are living with food allergies? Who is getting them and, more important, *why*? Which foods are people reacting to and, again more important, *why*? After decades of eating a certain food with no problem, how does an adult suddenly develop a severe allergy to it? What triggers this switch to suddenly turn on? Are reactions to some foods more severe than others? What is the difference between a food allergy and a food intolerance or "sensitivity" as many call it? How many people think they have food allergies but are suffering from one or more of those "masqueraders"? And whether we're dealing with a bona fide food allergy or masquerader, what are the best methods for diagnosing, treating, and managing these conditions? How do they impact both families and communities and what can we do to help them with daily challenges? Can we find treatments? Cures? And will those treatments and potential cures work for everyone and be equally accessible?

After gathering as much information as I could about food allergy, I noticed that fundamental data—such as the overall number of people in the US currently living with a food allergy—were entirely unknown. Understanding the gravity of the disease nationwide was the first critical step to making a difference for affected families, so I connected with a team of passionate researchers and supporters, and we got to work. We grew and built the Center for Food Allergy & Asthma Research (CFAAR) at Northwestern University Feinberg School of Medicine and Ann & Robert H. Lurie Children's Hospital of Chicago to look at allergic conditions from clinical, epidemiological, and community-facing lenses, and understand the public health impact of food allergy in the United States.

In 2011, my team and I surveyed a little more than forty thousand Americans and determined that 8 percent of children (1 in 13) have a food allergy, which equates to about two children in every classroom. The most commonly reported food allergens were peanuts, tree nuts, milk, eggs, shellfish, finfish, wheat, soy, and sesame—all very common foods in the American diet. As food allergy became a more widely discussed public health epidemic in the following years, we decided to redistribute this survey to parents of another 40,000 US children. However, at the same time, we also collected data from a sample of over forty thousand adults and asked them about their own food allergies. The results, as you may have read about, were shocking.

We used to think that food allergies almost always started early in life. However, our team's 2019 study with colleagues dispelled that notion and further complicated the mystery. Perhaps most surprising was finding that almost half of the adults with food allergies in our investigation had some in childhood but went on to develop additional allergies in adulthood, and about a quarter of them developed a food allergy seemingly out of the blue, as an adult. Again, what was the trigger that suddenly turned this switch on? This was no longer just a childhood problem.

The data are becoming clear: living with a food allergy or a masquerader can meaningfully reduce quality of life, impose substantial economic burden, limit one's dietary choices, and result in life-threatening reactions for the millions of Americans living it—a quadruple threat. This set of circumstances has been a regular topic of conversation for me at social gatherings for years now. Once I tell people what I do for a living, the floodgates open, and I soon find myself (happily and enthusiastically) inundated with questions and addressing confusion, curiosity, and anxiety. You may have also noticed that adverse food reactions are increasingly common dinner conversation. If you randomly asked your guests at a large gathering whether anyone has a food allergy, intolerance, or a related condition, you'll probably see many hands go up. Some of the culprits will sound typical, such as peanuts and tree nuts; some may surprise you: lobster, peas, mushrooms, salmon, tofu, or even red meat. And my bet is some of your guests will find it hard to define the difference between a food allergy and intolerance. They will use the terms liberally and interchangeably.

Everybody has an anecdote about when they first discovered their food condition. As someone working to promote public health, I find it fun and informative to discuss these patients' theories about how their food conditions came to be. Many times, these theories revolve around how different the world is now compared to when they were growing up:

> "When I was little, I had a PB&J every day at school! I can't believe peanuts aren't even allowed in classrooms anymore!"

"It has to be how the food is prepared."

"Overly processed foods with fillers, preservatives, GMO, refined ingredients, and additives are confusing our body."

"It's how we're farming today. Mass production with harmful
agrochemicals, right?"

"Baby foods are too commercialized today. My mother made
all my food from scratch when I was a baby—it didn't come
from a packaged box or jar."

"Americans are too clean; we need to start playing in the dirt
more so we keep our immune system charged and don't
develop allergies."

"We live in a toxic soup of chemicals. The stuff we're exposed
to and put in our body confuses it and turns our immune
system against us."

While some of these theories are being explored scientifically, the
truth is you can develop a genuine allergy, intolerance, or other masquerader to almost any food at any point in your lifetime, and we're
still hard at work trying to figure out exactly why and how to prevent them. The trauma of that first experience with a food allergy,
whether at age one, three, thirty-three, or sixty-three, can be equally
as upsetting and life changing. The good news is the future is bright
in our quest to prevent and treat food allergy, as well as further determine the relationships among allergy, intolerance, and other food
conditions.

Aside from the top nine food allergy culprits commonly discussed,
you'll increasingly hear people talking about their symptoms from a
variety of other foods, such as gluten, milk/dairy, fermented foods, or
certain kinds of herbs and spices, additives, dyes, preservatives, fresh
fruits, and vegetables. Gluten and dairy trigger severe gastrointestinal
distress; fruit makes their mouth tingle; a milk shake gives them a really terrible stomachache; Cheddar cheese sparks migraines. Troubling
symptoms indeed, but these may actually be signs of food intolerance,

or a variety of other food-related conditions on the spectrum. These "masqueraders" can include celiac disease, gluten or lactose intolerance, pollen-food allergy syndrome, eosinophilic esophagitis (EoE), intolerance to sulfites and nitrates, food protein–induced enterocolitis syndrome (FPIES), and more, which we will dive into deeper later in the book. It's important to distinguish between food reactions that recruit the immune system and those masqueraders that do not, or at least not in any life-threatening way.

At our research center, we are also hard at work trying to alleviate this confusion across the spectrum between food allergies and these other food-related conditions. I know the plethora of terms including "allergy," "intolerance," and "sensitivities" can be so baffling, so I'm here to help clarify these definitions. I realize that the term *food sensitivity* is used a lot in everyday conversations (e.g., "I'm sensitive to dairy, egg, and wheat."), but it's not a term well defined by the medical community. The National Institute of Allergy and Infectious Diseases (NIAID) only distinguishes "allergies" and "intolerances" so we'll stick with those terms as much as possible and, when appropriate, I'll call out differing language, some of which is more familiar to people.

Part of the goal of this book is to establish important distinctions, arrive at a universal vocabulary, and help people manage all types of food conditions. One of the biggest challenges of conducting food allergy research is that when my medical colleagues and I talk about "food allergy," we typically have the same disease in mind: an immediate, immune-based allergic response to a particular food that usually occurs within two hours. However, among the general public, the term "food allergy" is often used to refer to a wide variety of food-related conditions, many of which are not actually allergies. This confusion is understandable, particularly since some foods can be triggers of both allergic and nonallergic responses, and some patients can simultaneously harbor allergic and nonallergic food-related conditions.

There are plenty of gray areas to blur the conversation when it comes to food allergy. One good example is cow's milk, which is both the most common food allergy among US infants, and one of the most common food intolerances: two distinct conditions. While both can result in very unpleasant gastrointestinal symptoms, cow's milk intolerance (lactose intolerance) is caused by a missing enzyme (lactase) in the gut—not an immune response to the proteins in cow's milk. Consequently, these two conditions are treated very differently. For example, many patients with milk intolerance can consume small amounts of cow's milk without adverse effects so long as they first take a medicine containing their missing lactase enzyme to aid digestion. In contrast, there is no comparable over-the-counter treatment allowing milk-allergic patients to safely consume milk in any quantity, which is why strict allergen avoidance is so important.

Another gray area is wheat and its gluten component shared with other cereal grains. When patients experience adverse symptoms after eating wheat or gluten, they may be caused by food allergy to wheat proteins, gluten intolerance in celiac disease, or something else. Despite a shared trigger (eating wheat/gluten), each of these conditions requires different clinical testing, management, and treatment. Just that term alone, "gluten sensitivity," stirs a lot of confusion and misunderstanding that we'll explore.

In light of all the similarities between the symptoms and triggers of food allergies and these other food-related conditions, it is not surprising that so many people think that they have a food allergy. As I already mentioned, our 2019 study showed that nearly 1 in 5 American adults told us they believed they were currently allergic to at least one food. But after carefully examining their allergic reaction history and organ symptoms involved in their reactions, we determined that about 1 in 10 American adults has a convincing IgE-mediated food allergy (I'll explain what that means in detail later). It's abundantly clear that millions of Americans are still experiencing symptoms after eating specific foods and thus still suffer similar day-to-day stress and anxiety associated with avoiding suspected foods. Therefore, the number of people adversely affected by a food-related condition in the US is probably closer to ninety million! And *that's* a lot of people.

Additionally, only half of the adults reporting a convincing food allergy received a physician diagnosis. I know as adults we don't always take as good care of ourselves as we do our kids and often avoid going to the doctor unless we think it's absolutely essential. But it is really important for adults with suspected food allergies to consult a physician to truly understand what food-related condition they have and not unnecessarily remove foods from the diet. Moreover, consulting a physician can help you learn and implement the latest, most effective strategies for managing your food condition, since there are a rapidly growing number of medications and potential treatments.

Food Without Fear provides the facts and guidance to understand food allergies and other food-related conditions to help those affected by them to live confidently and safely. We're going to tackle the latest science, unpack hidden links between seemingly different sources of dysfunction in the body, and go so far as to reveal surprisingly powerful relationships between gut health and allergies. We'll answer the question that millions of people often face when they reach the end of the road with allergy testing: *If it's not an allergy and I still have symptoms, then what is it?* Perhaps nothing is more frustrating and psychologically deflating than suffering with no proper diagnosis. And you don't want to be told that it's "all in your head."

You'll find a blend of science distilled down to meaningful terms and practical takeaways. I realize that each individual comes to this book with their own unique set of circumstances, conditions, and personal health risk factors, but there are universal concepts and lessons to learn, as well as strategies to implement. Each chapter ends with Fearless Facts, a cheat sheet of sorts that summarizes the chapter's main ideas for easy reading and implementation of the knowledge. Not every piece of information may be relevant for you, but having a full grasp of the details that comprise this spectrum will ultimately help and empower you. My hope is that by understanding the spectrum of food-related conditions and how to manage them, you can lead a full, engaging, vibrant life that doesn't feel restricted or bound. I also aim to equip educators, health-care providers, and regulators with the crucial information they need to make their contribution in effecting positive change. In the chapters ahead, we're going to start by addressing the biggest question of all: Why? Why has the twenty-first century given us staggering advances in technology and medicine, yet when it comes to food-related conditions, we are witnessing a climb in cases and struggling to combat the biological blaze? What factors contribute to this epidemic that has such a wide and varied spectrum?

After a thorough look at what is driving the trend, we'll turn to what we can—and should—do about it. This includes in-depth conversations about evidence-based "best practices" for testing, diagnosing, treating, and managing food-related conditions across the entire spectrum (as well as my own framework of **Identify and Empower; Treat; Manage and Prevent; and Thrive**); guidance for parents, caregivers, and educators; support for addressing food-related conditions in adulthood, especially if they are new and unexpected; and insights about what we can do as a society to turn this epidemic around and snuff out the fire. The end result? Better health and wellness for everyone. Deliverance from fear of food. A more liberated life. Food freedom!

You may have heard about such revolutionary treatments as oral immunotherapy, an emerging practice in medicine to help people manage their food allergy and "reengineer" their bodies so they can tolerate a specific amount of their food allergen to reduce dangerous allergic reactions. It's based on the same incredible science that helps cancer patients tweak their immune systems to fight the rogue cells. Just as immunotherapy increasingly will be curative in the cancer world, thanks to the advancement of this technology coupled with an individualized approach to each patient's type of cancer and genomics (what's called precision medicine), so too can immunotherapy and precision medicine combined change the food allergy landscape.

Other treatments, including vaccines, patch desensitization, and biologic therapies are also coming into play. Who is a good candidate for these treatments and how do they work? Are they as promising as they sound? In 2020, the US Food and Drug Administration (FDA) approved the first peanut allergy "treatment" for children. But will it be our long-term solution for the one million kids who live with peanut allergy, of which only 1 in 5 children are likely to naturally outgrow? These are important questions to address. Each chapter will include wisdom not only from my own research but also from other scientists and specialists in this large and expanding field. I travel the world speaking and educating others about this explosive subject, and as you'll later see, there's a lot we can learn by looking at other parts of the world where these problems barely exist or, conversely, as they do in the United States, affect millions. Hope is on the horizon.

Before we venture forward, I want to share one of my favorite quotes from Maya Angelou, and my reason for writing this book: "When you learn, teach. When you get, give." I've learned a lot throughout my career and wanted to share that knowledge with you. Also, your purchase of this book will be part of giving back, as a portion of the proceeds will be donated to help deliver food to those in need. In this time of Covid-19 we have seen so many waiting in long lines for food and our intention is to help get people "food without fear." So, please now join me on this journey to remove the fear and to make food our friend again!

TEST YOUR FOOD IQ

How much do you know about food allergies? Find out using the following true/false quiz. Don't think too much about each question; answer as best you can (you're not being scored). The answers are on page xxi. By the end of the book, you'll have a full understanding about these topics.

1. Using hand-sanitizing gels (e.g., Purell) is an effective way to remove food allergens from one's hands. T/F

2. An antihistamine such as Benadryl should be given first for a serious allergic reaction. T/F

3. Food allergies are rare, impacting 1 in 100 people in the US. T/F

4. Food allergies and intolerances/sensitivities develop only in childhood. T/F

5. A reaction to pollenlike proteins in certain raw fruits and vegetables that triggers itchiness or swelling of the mouth, face, lip, tongue, and throat is an oral allergy syndrome. T/F

6. Reactions to foods, be they allergies or intolerances, are less common among patients identifying as Black or African American compared to their peers who identify as white. T/F

7. Infants most commonly develop hives or vomiting when experiencing a food allergy reaction to a new food. T/F

8. Most cases of bloating and gassiness caused by consuming milk or wheat (gluten) are probably a food allergy. T/F

9. Eczema in babies is a risk factor for the development of food allergies. T/F

10. Someone who gets food stuck in their esophagus could have a chronic inflammatory disease of the esophagus called eosinophilic esophagitis (EoE). T/F

11. A pregnant woman should avoid eating peanuts or introducing them to her future child too early. T/F

12. Precautionary allergen labels, such as "May contain" labels, are strictly regulated by the FDA. T/F

13. Food allergies are more common among people who live in rural areas than among city dwellers. T/F

14. People with sulfite intolerance do not need to avoid sulfa-based antibiotics. T/F

15. Food sensitivity tests you can buy online and in pharmacies are very useful in identifying problematic foods you should avoid. T/F

16. Typical Western diets can adversely affect your immune system and inflammation pathways. T/F

17. If you have a food allergy or food-related condition, the reaction will always occur within minutes. T/F

18. It is recommended that people with an intolerance to MSG need to carry an epinephrine auto-injector at all times. T/F

19. Testing IgG antibody levels in the blood to exposure to multiple foods (usually 90 to 100 foods with a single panel test) can help you definitively identify food allergies and intolerances. T/F

20. Reactions to food never change; you're stuck with them for life. T/F

Answers.

1. False	11. False
2. False	12. False
3. False	13. False
4. False	14. True
5. True	15. False
6. False	16. True
7. True	17. False
8. False	18. False
9. True	19. False
10. True	20. False

DECODING YOUR FOOD REACTIONS
The Questionnaire

I F I HAD TO OFFER A FIRST BIG STEP IN SOLVING YOUR FOOD REACTIONS, IT would be this: Get to know them. Ending or managing them begins with you. Solving food reactions is partly science and partly art. Although we have lots of high-tech tools available to us in medicine, diagnosing food reactions is not as absolute and straightforward as many people imagine. I research food allergies, so you can imagine how surprised I was to find that so many US adults—one in five—reported a "food allergy." We quickly understood how much confusion there is around food conditions. In this book, I want to help people understand what they have, what may cause it, what happens in their body, and how to properly diagnose, manage, and even treat it.

Unfortunately, unless you have a very easily diagnosable condition that's not complicated by another health challenge, figuring out a root cause of a food reaction can be complex and immensely vexing. So, the more you can contribute to the story of your reactions, the more you can shift your experience to one that's less reliant on art and pseudoscience and more based on data-driven science.

As a useful exercise at the start of the book, which will equip you with the information you need to decode your own unique condition(s), use the following checklist to organize your thoughts and personal information. This questionnaire is designed to help you prepare for a doctor's visit, giving you clues to what to discuss. I also realize you want to be told what to do as soon as possible, and even though you'll find much to consider throughout this book, the following questions will provide you with concepts to think about as you read further and apply these ideas to your life. Your answers will help you get the most out of this book and find a solution sooner rather than later.

Directions: Answer as many of the following questions that apply to you (or a loved one who has a food-related concern) and bring this checklist with you to your/their doctor. Add additional notes where necessary. You'll find this online at www .foodwithoutfearbook.com to download as well.

These questions outline aspects of your/their medical history and experiences that are important for a health-care provider to consider when evaluating a food-related condition.

What do you hope to achieve by better understanding where you fall on the spectrum of adverse food reactions?

What foods give you trouble? List all, whether they are whole foods (e.g., peaches and eggs), whole categories of foods (e.g., dairy, shellfish), or single ingredients often mixed with other ingredients (e.g., gluten, sulfites, sugar):

1.
2.
3.
4.

Family history:

CONDITION	MOM	DAD	SIBLING(S)
Eczema			
Asthma			
Hay fever			
Food allergy			
Autoimmune disease			
Celiac disease			

Have you ever been diagnosed with any other health condition?
- ❏ Allergic conditions (e.g., eczema, hay fever, asthma)
- ❏ Metabolic conditions (e.g., insulin resistance, diabetes)
- ❏ Digestive disorders (e.g., irritable bowel syndrome, inflammatory bowel disease [Crohn's or ulcerative colitis], gastroesophageal reflux disease [GERD])
- ❏ Autoimmune conditions (e.g., celiac disease, chronic fatigue, psoriasis, fibromyalgia, Hashimoto's thyroiditis, rheumatoid arthritis)
- ❏ Other (e.g., depression, serious infections)

Do you take any medications, vitamins, or supplements, including those unrelated to any food condition?
- ❏ Yes (if so, list . . .)
- ❏ No

Environmental history:

How old is your primary residence?

How long have you lived there?

Is there carpeting in this home? Y/N

Has there been water damage? Y/N

Are there any pets? Y/N

For each of those foods that you listed as causing you trouble:

What are your main symptoms? (check all that apply)

- ❑ Hives
- ❑ Rashes, itchy skin
- ❑ Coughing, wheezing, short of breath, trouble breathing
- ❑ Chest pain
- ❑ Sneezing
- ❑ Watery or red eyes
- ❑ Runny or stuffy nose
- ❑ Stomach pain, cramping, bloating, gas, intestinal distress
- ❑ Heartburn, acid reflux
- ❑ Diarrhea or constipation
- ❑ Nausea
- ❑ Vomiting
- ❑ Throat tightening
- ❑ Trouble swallowing
- ❑ Food "feeling stuck"
- ❑ Tingling or itching in the mouth or on the lips
- ❑ Dizziness, lightheadedness
- ❑ Sense of impending doom
- ❑ Swelling of your face, tongue, throat, abdomen, or arms and legs
- ❑ Blood in stools
- ❑ Unexplained weight gain or loss
- ❑ Eczema
- ❑ Headaches, migraines
- ❑ Joint pain
- ❑ Brain fog, inability to focus or concentrate
- ❑ Irritability or nervousness
- ❑ Lethargy, malaise
- ❑ Anxiety around food
- ❑ Other _____

At what age did you first experience food-related symptoms?

When you've had a reaction to this food, when did the reaction start?
- ❏ Within 15 minutes of eating the food
- ❏ Between 15 minutes to 2 hours
- ❏ >2 hours to 24 hours
- ❏ More than 24 hours
- ❏ I don't know

Have you ever been tested or in any way evaluated for any food allergy or sensitivity/intolerance?*
- ❏ Yes, by a medical professional (If so, what type of clinician? What was diagnosed? What was recommended to manage, treat, and prevent?)
- ❏ Yes, using a store-bought or mail-order (over-the-counter) sensitivity kit (If so, what were the results?)
- ❏ No

*Be sure to bring any test results to your doctor's appointment.

Have you ever tried a specific diet to treat your condition?
- ❏ Yes, and my symptoms improved (please describe . . .)
- ❏ Yes, and my symptoms worsened (please describe . . .)
- ❏ Yes, and I saw no change (please describe . . .)
- ❏ No

Have you tried any additional (nondietary) therapies to control symptoms, including prescribed drugs or over-the-counter treatments?
- ❏ Yes, and my symptoms improved (please describe . . .)
- ❏ Yes, and my symptoms worsened (please describe . . .)
- ❏ Yes, and I saw no change (please describe . . .)
- ❏ No

Do certain activities or moments in your life seem to make your reactions worse, such as exercise, drinking alcohol, certain medications, menstrual period, travel, periods of acute stress?

❑ Yes (please describe . . .)
❑ No
❑ I don't know

Information is power. The more you can track your experience, the more information you have to use in identifying, managing, treating, and ultimately gaining control of your condition(s) and preventing future episodes. Later in the book, I'll present an acronym—STOP—that will further help you arrive at solutions. Here's a quick preview:

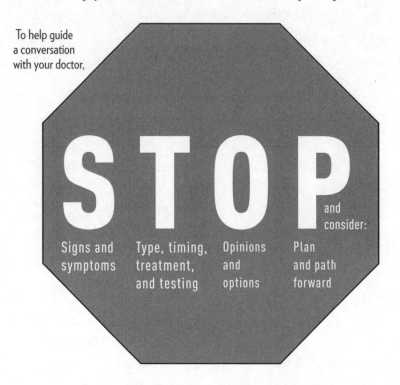

Let's first gain a full understanding of food reactions and then you'll have the information you need to chart your path to food freedom.

WHAT IS YOUR STORY?

I love shellfish and have had them all my life. About a year ago at the age of 31, I had shellfish and my throat felt funny and I got a few hives on my neck and was itching. It is so hard to avoid and I try, but occasionally when I have some I have similar symptoms.

I have been allergic to peanuts and walnuts all my life. I am now an adult and have mild symptoms with tingling in my mouth and sometimes a rash to many more foods, including tomatoes, avocados, and mangoes. I have not had nuts and have not had a reaction for a long time but have not gone to an allergist about these foods since I was a kid.

I have a 15-year-old child with sesame and peanut allergies. It is challenging avoiding the foods and he had a recent anaphylactic reaction for which we gave epinephrine and rushed him to the emergency department, where he had to get another round of epi and oxygen and albuterol with steroids, as he also has asthma. I really want him to get treatment before going to college. I want him to be able to go out with his friends without worrying about a reaction.

In my midtwenties, I started to restrict many foods from my diet—chiefly gluten, wheat, dairy, most fruits, and all legumes, nuts, and seeds—under _the thinking that I was either sensitive or allergic to these foods. I had chronic GI issues (gas, bloating, diarrhea, constipation), could not control my weight, and would get a migraine at least once a month. Now forty, I further restrict certain foods and struggle with an eating disorder. I wonder what foods are really giving me trouble and if I'm even "allergic" to anything or whether it's all in my head._

I have a 6-month-old infant with eczema. I tried starting her on peanuts by mixing peanut butter and water, and the first time, she was fine. The second time, she got a rash around her mouth. I was worried she had an allergy to it and stopped feeding it to her.

When I hit menopause, my body changed so much that no matter what diet I tried to gain control of my weight (and sanity), I failed. I also felt chronically sluggish with stomach discomfort, brain fog, and no motivation to work out. So, I bought one of those at-home food sensitivity kits that you see advertised online or in the drugstore and found out, somewhat to my shock, that I'm allergic to many foods I've been eating forever. But then a friend said I'm probably not really allergic and to consider seeing a gastroenterologist and dietitian in addition to an allergist to figure this out.

I am a 50-year-old woman who has developed "adult acne." I hate it. I also have more bloating, diarrhea, abdominal pain, constipation, bad breath, and acid reflux than ever before. Are they connected? It doesn't help that I'm under a lot of stress and eat poorly due to my demanding job and family life. I don't know what's causing my problems, but I need to fix this fast.

Although your story is unique to you, with the increase in food allergies and related conditions, your story is also part of a shared experience with many others. I hope to provide answers and guidance throughout this book for you and hope you continue to share your story. Go to www.foodwithoutfearbook.com to join our community.

PART I

THE FOOD REACTION SPECTRUM

Where Are You?

one

BODY BACKLASH

The Surprising Rise of Reactions to Food in the 21st Century and the Search for Answers

WHEN JAMISON VULOPAS ("JJ") WAS TWO YEARS OLD, HE CONSUMED A seemingly innocuous sour cream and onion potato chip made with milk products—and had the first major reaction that sent his body into a spiral of severe symptoms. Although he eventually outgrew an allergy to peanuts (a legume) and eggs, he's been allergic to milk and tree nuts his entire life. As a young boy, he learned how to deal with his allergies with the help of his parents who kept the house safe and were extraprotective of him. But it wasn't easy. By the time he entered middle school, JJ decided he would no longer be defined—or confined—by his allergies. He didn't want to be "that food allergy kid" only known for being "the one who can't drink milk or eat nuts." It was time to come out of his emotional shell, take full ownership of his allergies, and turn them into a positive attribute.

And that he did, becoming class president his senior year in high school and moving on to the University of Pennsylvania, where he wrote his first book, *Land of Not*, to teach kids with allergies how to frame their condition in their lives and have a healthy relationship with it. The book soon became a message not just for kids with allergies, but for all children who think negatively about themselves and feel "less than" their peers. Its core message is simple: Do what you love. Embrace what you've got. You are who you are. Not who you're not. Live in the land of CAN. Today, JJ is a young adult with his college degree who is navigating the world of finance in New York City and, when he has time, maintaining a website and writing about health, safety, and empowerment books based around the "can" philosophy.

I met JJ in 2018 at a food allergy conference, when he reached out to me and gave me his amazing book. I was immediately impressed with his passion, talent, and desire to make an impact. About a year later, my daughter, who also has food allergies, cowrote another book with JJ for schools to introduce and discuss food allergies with their students. JJ is the perfect example of what it can be like for kids to grow up feeling insecure about their food allergies and how they can eventually find a way to become their own best advocate and gain skills to protect themselves and turn their situation into a net positive. You can learn to appreciate the condition and educate others. I trust JJ will have some remarkable achievements in his life and share his hard-won experience with the world. Although he has to think about his food allergy every day, it no longer is a source of fear and trepidation. He's starting oral immunotherapy (see Chapter 7) for his allergens, but he is thriving despite his limitations and enjoying life to the fullest. Like other young adults who have been living with food allergies most of their life, he has learned how to be fully engaged no matter where he is—at home, at work, out with friends, and throughout his community (including his online one at www.thelandofcan.com).

When my group asked young adults what positive attributes they got from their food allergies, the top responses were an improved ability to advocate for themselves and greater empathy for others. JJ fully embodies these admirable traits, which any parents would hope for in their children. It also reflects an attitude that anyone—regardless of age—would do well to adopt: by being aware and empowered with the right knowledge, advocating for ourselves and having empathy for others, we can live fearlessly with any type of food-related condition across the entire spectrum.

THE SCOPE OF THIS 21ST-CENTURY EPIDEMIC

As I noted in the Introduction, 2011 was a game changer in my field when my team at the Center for Food Allergy & Asthma Research (CFAAR) published, in the journal *Pediatrics*, the most comprehensive and widely cited estimate to date of the prevalence and severity of childhood food allergy in the US. Additionally, updated data published in 2018 also shined a light on the relationship between food allergies and food intolerances. This was followed by our much publicized 2019 publication in the *Journal of the American Medical Association Network Open* that spotlighted the surprising food allergy phenomenon among adults.

Every three minutes, a food allergy reaction sends someone in the US to the emergency room. Each year in this country, at least one million patients receive emergency medical care for allergic reactions to food. Our data estimate that up to 32 million Americans have food allergies, including 6 million children under age eighteen (about 8 percent of the pediatric population). As a reminder, that's 1 in 13 children, or roughly two in every classroom and 1 in 10 adults. The Centers for Disease Control and Prevention (CDC) report that the prevalence of food allergy in children increased by 50 percent between 1997 and 2011. About 40 percent of children with a food allergy will experience a severe reaction. People can be allergic to any food, but the top nine food allergens are peanuts, milk, shellfish, tree nuts, eggs, finfish, wheat, soy, and sesame.

Recent numbers published by my colleagues and I show that about 40 percent of children with food allergies are allergic to more than one food. Importantly, food allergies are costly both financially and emotionally. My research has estimated that American families spend nearly $25 billion annually caring for children with food allergies (special diets and medications, changing jobs and even place of living to be close to the right medical care; a little more than $4,000 per year is the average additional amount incurred by a family with a child with food allergy). There are social tolls as well: About 1 in 3 children with food allergy report being bullied as a result. Adults with food allergies can also suffer emotional and financial expenses, not to mention major impairments to their quality of life. And as I already mentioned, while many food allergies do typically develop in the first few years of a person's life, nearly half of more than twenty-six million American adults (about 10 percent of all adults) with a food allergy developed at least one allergy *after the age of eighteen*. Of those twenty-six million American adults, 25 percent had their very first food allergy reaction as an adult.

Although acute and severe reactions that impact multiple organ systems and cause such symptoms as trouble breathing, a drop in blood pressure, and vomiting are rare, between 2007 and 2016, health claims for this frightening condition, called anaphylaxis, went up 883 percent among nineteen- to thirty-year-olds. Food allergy is one of the most common causes of anaphylaxis and accounts for 30 to 50 percent of all anaphylaxis cases and up to 81 percent of anaphylaxis cases in children. Over 50 percent of children and adults with food allergy reported experiencing an allergic reaction in the past year, with 1 in 4 requiring epinephrine. Additionally, 1 in 5 children with food allergy were seen in the emergency department in the past year for a food allergic reaction.

However, this is not just an American epidemic. Current global trends show that the number of people reacting to foods is increasing at an alarming rate, particularly in developed countries. In Australia, 1 in 10 infants suffers from a food allergy, which is the highest prevalence of food allergy ever reported on the planet. Worldwide, we are seeing food allergies increasing. On my travels to Australia, India, and Europe, I've spoken to many people about the rise in food allergies and related food conditions, such as intolerances and what many refer to as "sensitivities," which again are technically not allergies or allergic disorders. But people confuse the terms—they don't understand what's going on in their body and how they can manage their symptoms. Around 20 percent of the US population think they may have a "food allergy," but as previously called out, about half of those folks may not have an immune-mediated food allergy and instead suffer from another food-related condition, such as an intolerance. Moreover, only 5 percent are getting a doctor's diagnosis, and the other 15 percent are avoiding foods without truly knowing what could be happening.

What exactly is a true "food allergy"? By definition, a food allergy is a medical condition in which exposure to a food consistently triggers a harmful immune response. That's a key point to remember: the body's natural defense system—the immune system—is involved; it awakens as though it's responding to a serious invader. The immune response, called an allergic reaction, occurs because the immune system treats certain proteins in the food as a threat rather than recognizing them as the harmless nutrients they are. The proteins that trigger the reaction are called allergens. The symptoms of an allergic reaction to food can range from mild (itchy mouth, a few hives) to severe (throat tightening or swelling, difficulty breathing, drop in blood pressure). Allergic reactions are not uniform; they affect people differently, range in severity, and manifest in myriad bodily symptoms depending on the type of reaction, the amount of food consumed, and the person affected. The most dangerous and severe reaction is anaphylaxis. Several types of reactions can occur in the same individual and a previous mild reaction doesn't always mean future reactions will be mild.

The Top 9 Food Allergens

- Peanuts
- Tree Nuts (e.g., walnuts, pecans, almonds, cashews, hazelnuts, Brazil nuts, pistachios, macadamia nuts)
- Milk
- Egg
- Shellfish (e.g., lobster, shrimp, crab, clams, mussels, oysters)
- Finfish (e.g., salmon, cod, halibut, catfish)
- Soy
- Wheat
- Sesame

Note: the word *nut* is often used broadly and does not always refer to a true tree nut. Macadamia nuts and pine nuts, for example, are both seeds. Coconut is a fruit, although the FDA labels coconut as a tree nut. Similarly, nutmeg, water chestnut, butternut squash, and shea nuts are not tree nuts and, like coconut, are generally well tolerated by tree nut–allergic individuals. Also note that although 30 percent of individuals allergic to peanuts are also allergic to at least one tree nut, having a tree nut allergy does not necessarily mean the person is allergic to peanuts. Tree nuts are also unique, and people can be allergic to some and eat others. Recent research is also finding certain tree nuts, such as cashew and pistachio, and walnut and pecan, run together. People with a tree nut allergy can usually consume seeds without difficulty, such as sesame, sunflower, and pumpkin.

Common Offenders for Food Intolerances

dairy	amines**	monosodium glutamate (MSG)
gluten	sulfites	food dyes
caffeine	fructose	
salicylates*	alcohol	

*Salicylates are naturally occurring compounds in plants (fruits and vegetables).

**Amines are products of protein breakdown in food. They are high in cheese, chocolate, wine, beer, yeast extracts, and fish products. They are also found in certain fruits and vegetables (e.g., bananas, avocados, tomatoes, and broad beans).

ALLERGIES VS. INTOLERANCES

Before we do a deep dive into the world of food allergies and intolerances, let's clearly define the difference. They are not the same, though people routinely use these terms interchangeably (being "lactose intolerant," for example, is not a milk allergy). According to the National Institute of Allergy and Infectious Diseases (NIAID), a food allergy is defined as "an adverse health effect arising from a specific immune response that occurs reproducibly on exposure to a given food" and food intolerance as reproducible adverse reactions to food that *do not have an established or likely immunologic mechanism*. As previously noted, the term *sensitivity* is commonly used, but it's not clearly defined in the medical literature. So, for the purpose of this book and in the name of accuracy, we will use *intolerance* to include what is commonly referred to as a sensitivity.

And therein lies the key difference between a specific immune system response (allergy) and a digestive system or metabolic response (intolerance) whose symptoms are induced by other pathways. **But signs and symptoms can often overlap, and timing of symptoms as well**, sometimes making a correct diagnosis feel like a puzzle to figure out. The major line that separates these two large categories of food issues is whether the immune system is involved—and how so. Food allergies engage the immune system—they are immune-mediated reactions to food. As we'll explore in the next chapter, the most common is an immunoglobulin E (IgE)–mediated reaction.

An IgE-mediated reaction is generally an immediate reaction to a food caused by allergic antibodies known as IgE. People who are allergic to certain triggers, such as peanut, birch pollen, or dust mites, have specific IgE antibodies that react only to those specific triggers. When an allergic person is exposed to their allergen, these allergens travel to cells (e.g., mast cells), which have IgE antibodies on their surface that specifically recognize the allergens, and these cells then release chemicals (e.g., histamine), which cause an allergic reaction.

There are also non-IgE mediated food allergies that occur when other parts of the immune system are activated apart from IgE antibodies. An example of a non-IgE-mediated immune reaction that was once very rare but is now on the rise is food protein–induced enterocolitis syndrome (FPIES, pronounced "F-pies"). This syndrome, which is most commonly triggered by grains (e.g., wheat, rice, oats, barley) and dairy (e.g., cow's milk), usually starts during infancy and is often outgrown by age two, though it can occur in older children and adults as well. The symptoms of non-IgE allergic reactions are typically delayed by several hours following ingestion and take place primarily in the gastrointestinal tract. They most commonly include forceful vomiting, diarrhea, and/or bloating. FPIES in particular is known for characteristically violent vomiting, which often leads parents of kids who suddenly experience these symptoms to think "stomach bug," until symptoms recur upon repeated exposure to the trigger food. FPIES reactions can be severe and lead to serious medical complications from the profuse vomiting, diarrhea, and other symptoms. A recent review study concluded: "Although there have been no reported cases of fatality from FPIES, acute reactions can induce hypotension and hypothermia."

Similarly, food protein–induced allergic proctocolitis (FPIAP), which is also rare but increasingly diagnosed, typically starts in the first few months of life and is manifested with rectal bleeding in otherwise healthy infants. This is likely due to a reaction to cow's milk consumed by the mother if breastfeeding or by the infant directly to the milk if formula fed. And, like FPIES, FPIAP tends to go away on its own over time, but it's one of the major causes of colitis (inflammation of the colon) during infancy. Even rarer is food-induced pulmonary hemosiderosis (a.k.a. Heiner syndrome, or cow's milk hypersensitivity), which is a reaction to cow's milk that triggers pulmonary and other problems in children, such as respiratory tract infections, anemia, and pneumonia. This is the lesser-known and much rarer non-IgE-mediated food allergy of the bunch. To make matters even more complicated, there can be mixed IgE- and non-IgE-mediated reactions, as can be the case with eosinophilic esophagitis or eosinophilic gastroenteritis, but we'll get to those rare diagnoses later. For now, let's remember that in contrast to food allergy, food intolerances are not caused by an immune reaction to food.

Symptoms of Food Intolerances

Whereas symptoms of food allergies can involve any organ system with hives, swelling, itching, wheezing, trouble breathing and swallowing due to constriction of the throat and airways, dizziness, a weak pulse, vomiting, and stomach pain, food intolerances are frequently confined to digestive matters, such as bloating, diarrhea or constipation, nausea, stomach cramps, and gas. Unlike a true, IgE-mediated food allergy, these symptoms are generally less serious and typically do not lead to anaphylaxis.

Food sensitivities/intolerances result from a variety of circumstances, among them:

→ you have a dysregulation of the digestive tract where you may not have the right enzymes you need to digest a certain food and therefore have a metabolic food intolerance (e.g., people who are lactose intolerant cannot digest milk sugar because they lack lactase in the gut—again, it's not an allergic response to the proteins in cow's milk);

→ you are reacting to food additives or preservatives, such as MSG, artificial colors, nitrites, or sulfites (e.g., sulfites used to preserve dried fruit, canned goods, and wine can trigger asthma attacks in sensitive people);

→ you are reacting to chemicals found in what you've ingested, such as caffeine, amines (especially histamines naturally found in aged foods, such as certain wines, cheeses, and smoked or preserved meats), salicylates (a group of plant chemicals found naturally in many fruits, vegetables, nuts, coffee, juices, beer, and wine), or even drugs, such as aspirin (aspirin happens to be a compound from the salicylate family; foods containing salicylates can trigger symptoms in people who are sensitive to aspirin);

→ you have irritable bowel syndrome (IBS), which is a chronic condition that causes abdominal cramping, constipation, and diarrhea, and can also flare up upon ingestion of certain foods, but IBS is not a food allergy. It's one of many "other" conditions that must be diagnosed apart from a food allergy or intolerance; because its symptoms mimic those of food allergy or intolerance, this serious condition can remain "camouflaged" and take time to discover. Inflammatory bowel diseases (IBD), such as ulcerative colitis and Crohn's, also need to be distinguished and treated separately, though some of the dietary edits patients with these conditions make can be similar to managing food allergy and intolerances;

→ you have galactosemia ("galactose in the blood"), so you cannot digest the sugar carbohydrate galactose, which comes from lactose-containing foods (dairy and breast milk), legumes, and some fruits and vegetables; the galactose builds up in the blood and is life-threatening (this is a rare disorder caused by a genetic mutation and is discovered in infants usually through the newborn screening).

I should note that reactions to certain drugs can be on the spectrum as well. Some people have true, immune-mediated drug allergies (e.g., to penicillin, chemotherapy drugs) that can incite the immune system and lead to anaphylaxis, whereas others are merely sensitive to a drug's side effects or have a reaction that entails symptoms similar to a drug allergy but does not involve the immune system. This latter condition is called a nonallergic hypersensitivity reaction (a.k.a. a pseudoallergic drug reaction). Common examples include reactions to dyes used in imaging tests or opiates and nonsteroidal anti-inflammatory drugs (NSAIDS) for treating pain.

MORE THAN FOOD: OTHER TRIGGERS BESIDES FOOD CAN CAUSE ANAPHYLAXIS IN SOME PEOPLE

Common triggers include insect stings (e.g., bees, fire ants), drugs (e.g., antibiotics, nonsteroidal anti-inflammatory drugs, chemotherapy drugs), and natural rubber latex. As many as a quarter of cancer patients develop allergic reactions to chemotherapy drugs several rounds into treatment. People with an allergy to latex can have allergic reactions when eating certain foods. These include avocado, banana, chestnut, kiwifruit, passion fruit, plum, strawberry, and tomato. This is because some of the proteins in latex that cause latex allergy are also present in these fruits. Some can have reactions to exercise as well, but those usually occur in combination with the consumption of food within a certain time period (more on exercise-induced anaphylaxis shortly).

Although the mere thought of a certain food can make you queasy or sick to your stomach, this is neither a food allergy nor intolerance. Recurring stress or psychological factors can be to blame, and this is poorly understood (though anyone who has experienced food poisoning and thereafter had a distaste for that particular food knows that our relationship with food can be deeply experiential and emotional). Another category that falls under food sensitivity/intolerance is fairly new to the scene: FODMAPs.

FODMAPs ("fod-maps")

The abbreviation FODMAPs stands for "fermentable oligo-, di-, mono-saccharides and polyols." FODMAPs are a group of short-chain carbohydrates found naturally in many foods that can cause digestive distress. In people sensitive to these carbs, the FODMAPs are poorly absorbed by the small intestine and travel on to the large intestine where the naturally occurring gut bacteria consume them as fuel by breaking them down and "fermenting" them, a process that results in gas and bloating. These carbohydrates also have osmotic properties, meaning they draw water into the digestive system, causing diarrhea and discomfort. FODMAP intolerances are very common in people with irritable bowel syndrome (IBS); up to 86 percent of people diagnosed with IBS experience a reduction in digestive symptoms when following a low-FODMAP diet. Foods high in FODMAPs include apples, artichokes, broccoli, Brussels sprouts, onion, cauliflower, cabbage, milk, soft cheeses, honey, bread, beans and lentils, and beer.

Unlike most people with a food allergy, those with food intolerances are often able to eat small amounts of the offending food without trouble, or the severity of their symptoms may be proportional to the amount of each exposure. Or they can prevent a reaction; lactose intolerance, for instance, can be overcome at a meal with lactase enzyme pills (that provide the enzyme needed to digest the lactose in the milk product) or by choosing a lactose-free milk product. I've been to pizza joints that sell lactose-free cheese pizza and gluten-free crusts.

Speaking of gluten, I get asked about this now-infamous ingredient all the time. It can be confusing because so many people now feel "gluten sensitive." What does that mean?

The Stickiness in the Gluten Debate

In today's society, gluten has taken over as the top avoided food due to a myriad of possible food conditions associated with it. Gluten is a protein composite found in the grains wheat, barley, and rye. Gluten is not a single molecule; it's made up of two main groups of proteins, the glutenins and the gliadins. A person can be sensitive to either of these proteins or to one of the twelve different smaller units that make up gliadin. *Gluten* actually means "glue" in Latin, and is widely used in breads and doughs, as well as other processed foods (such as sauces) because of its powerful binding and stabilizing properties.

If you have celiac disease, you have neither a food intolerance nor an IgE-mediated food allergy, though the disease does have some features of a food allergy because it involves the immune system but not in exactly the same way. However, whereas in food allergy the target of the immune system is a food protein, in celiac disease the target of the immune system is the patient's own tissue. For this reason, celiac disease is known as an **autoimmune** (*auto* is Greek for "self") disorder. In particular, celiac disease is characterized by damage to the small intestine upon gluten ingestion; the gluten triggers an immune-based reaction that ultimately attacks the small intestine's lining and prevents it from absorbing some nutrients. Symptoms often include gastrointestinal issues (e.g., diarrhea, bloating, gas, nausea, vomiting, constipation, and weight loss) as well as those seemingly unrelated to the digestive system, such as joint pain, fatigue, anemia, skin rashes, mouth ulcers, and headaches. The inflammation and decreased absorption can also lead to weight loss, poor growth, bone loss, and neurological problems. This needs focused evaluation and follow-up by a gastroenterologist and other specialists for its many possible complications. Currently, the only treatment for celiac is a life-long gluten-free diet, which leads to resolution of symptoms and healing of the intestinal damage.

People with celiac disease are not at risk of anaphylaxis. More recently, scientists have recognized what's called *nonceliac gluten sensitivity* as a common problem whereby people have symptoms of gluten intolerance but not the intestinal damage that defines celiac disease. I should add that celiac disease affects about 1 percent of the population. It's largely genetically driven but can become active after surgery, pregnancy, childbirth, viral infection, or severe emotional stress. And it can present at any age, so even people who have eaten gluten without problems for decades can develop celiac disease. People who do not have celiac disease but feel better after they've gone on a gluten-free diet could owe their improved health to reducing irritation from gluten grains from an unidentified process or to nixing other problematic ingredients that often travel with gluten. Moreover, when you make any dietary change, you likely change other health behaviors that may contribute to improving symptoms. It's important to note, though, that there's much debate in this area and researchers are still learning more about gluten sensitivity.

To be clear, food allergies are caused by any of the proteins in wheat; celiac disease is caused by the gluten in wheat. Although we don't know the precise cause of IBS, we know that it can be triggered by certain foods, especially dairy products, citrus fruits, beans, cabbage, carbonated drinks, and wheat due to the fructans (a type of carbohydrate) found in wheat. We also know that changes in gut microbes may be playing an important role, as people with IBS tend to have different microbial compositions than their healthy counterparts.

As we'll explore in upcoming chapters, the strength and function of your microbiome—the collection of microbes that live with you inside and out—could have a role in whether you develop allergies and other food-related conditions. We'll explore more about this phenomenon in Chapter 4, as it further colors the spectrum of adverse food reactions.

IT'S COMPLICATED BUT SOLVABLE

Various myths swirl around the topic of allergies, many of which I hope I've already begun to debunk as I open your eyes up to the scope—and pervasiveness—of the problem. Although diagnosing food allergies can be challenging, pinpointing food intolerances often presents an even greater challenge because so many symptoms can overlap and mimic a variety of other conditions, and the reactions can be delayed—further complicating the picture. Once you begin to feel the effects of a food intolerance, for example, hours could have passed since you ate a meal filled with a diverse array of ingredients. So, was it the soy or the MSG, the gluten or the FODMAPs? Later in the book, I'll give you some guidelines to follow in tracking down the culprit(s) and knowing what your next steps should be. Once you know where you stand on the spectrum, you will know which steps to take.

Speaking of the spectrum, I've mapped out what it looks like visually. The umbrella graphic on pages 18–19 will be something you'll want to come back to again and again as you read further. This shows most of the different adverse food reactions possible—from immediate, sometimes severe symptoms on the left to other food-related conditions that can often be masqueraders with delayed symptoms on the right. Use this as your guide.

A Little Help from My Friends

Denise and Dave Bunning are among my heroes in the food allergy community. They've been through it all over the past twenty-odd years and are now among the world's greatest advocates and donors to food allergy research and awareness. In the mid-1990s, when food allergies were barely on anyone's radar, these warrior parents were learning to cope with two young sons who suffered from life-threatening food allergies. One son was asthmatic as well as allergic to milk, eggs, and tree nuts; the other was allergic to milk, tree nuts, shellfish, finfish, and beef, and also was diagnosed with eosinophilic esophagitis ("EoE"). I'll discuss EoE in greater detail later, but in brief, EoE is characterized by an allergic reaction that causes inflammation of the esophagus. Although it's still considered a rare disease, it's increasingly diagnosed in children and adults, affecting an estimated 1 in 2,000 people.

For the Bunnings, learning to help manage their sons' allergies as they matured was a learn-as-you-go journey that inspired them to found organizations that would support the community, bring families together, raise awareness, and spur research. Denise cofounded MOCHA (Mothers of Children Having Allergies), a Chicago-based support group for food-allergic families; Dave co-founded the Food Allergy Project in 2005, which eventually combined with Food Allergy Research & Education (FARE; www.FoodAllergy.org). FARE is the world's leading nongovernmental organization engaged in food allergy advocacy and the largest private funder of food allergy research. It was formally referred to as the acronym but is now known simply as FARE, having expanded their mission to include the 85 million Americans who avoid the top 9 allergens due to food allergy and food intolerance, as well as the half billion people worldwide.

Both of Denise and Dave's sons are now thriving as young adults and have outgrown some of their allergies, but they still face the daily trials of managing their remaining food allergies amid traveling with demanding jobs and lots of meals eaten away from home.

Spectrum of

Immediate Symptoms

Anaphylaxis*
Impending doom
Low blood pressure/shock
Dizziness/light headedness
Hives

Facial swelling
Throat swelling/itchy mouth
Difficulty breathing/cough
Nasal congestion/runny nose
Vomiting
Diarrhea/cramping

Allergies**

Food allergy
Pollen-food allergy syndrome
   (PFAS), a.k.a. oral allergy
   syndrome (OAS)
Alpha-gal syndrome
Exercise-induced anaphylaxis

Mixed Reactions

Atopic dermatitis (eczema)
Eosinophilic esophagitis (EoE)
Eosinophilic gastrointestinal
   disorders (EGID)
Food Protein–induced
   enterocolitis syndrome
   (FPIES)

*Anaphylaxis reflects a constellation of symptoms, many of which are in the same "immediate" family list.

**While the immediate symptoms are more associated with allergic conditions, they are not exclusive to them (and vice versa with delayed reactions).

Adverse Food Reactions

Delayed Symptoms

Stomach cramping
Nausea/vomiting
Bloating/gas
Diarrhea
Constipation
Blood in stools

Headache/migraine
Eczema/rashes
Irritability/lethargy
Brain fog/forgetfulness
Weight loss or gain

Masqueraders

Milk, gluten, and other food
    sensitivities
Lactose intolerance
Chemical sensitivities (e.g.,
    caffeine, amines, sulfites,
    salicylates, alkaloids, MSG,
    alcohol)
Intolerance to food additives,
    dyes, preservatives
Intolerance to certain carbs (e.g.,
    fructose, sugar alcohols)
Allergic contact dermatitis
Gustatory rhinitis

Other Masqueraders

Gastro intestinal disorders
    (e.g., IBS, IBD)
Celiac disease
Gastroesophageal reflux disease
    (GERD)
Hiatal hernia
Food poisoning (e.g., salmonella,
    scombroid)
Intestinal infections
Food phobias/aversions
Eating disorders

When I asked Denise and Dave where they'd like to see the food allergy field in ten years, they both reiterated what I was already thinking: "In ten years," Dave said, "I would hope we would be transitioning from a world where anaphylaxis has been marginalized to a world that allows allergic individuals to openly eat food that they were previously allergic to. Moving the needle faster will require the pharmaceutical industry to join with physicians and the FDA to streamline the drug development process. Currently, each allergen is treated as a separate 'disease' when conducting research and going through the FDA. In my view, there needs to be a paradigm shift toward viewing food allergy as a disease, not a specific allergen. This will allow efficiencies with multiallergen clinical trials saving hundreds of millions in development costs."

For example, although a peanut allergy oral immunotherapy was recently approved by the FDA, using the exact same approach to treat another food, say almond, requires a completely separate series of clinical trials to test its safety, efficacy, and effectiveness. When you consider the fact that the average time it takes a therapy to go from filing an "Investigative New Drug" application to FDA approval is twelve years, addressing the burgeoning food allergy epidemic via such approaches is clearly not ideal.

"We all know," Denise said, "that food challenges are the current entry criteria for clinical trials. I'd like to hope that using a diagnostic that doesn't require triggering, and stopping, an allergic reaction will be developed and accepted as a replacement for food challenges. Not only would this new tool speed development of therapies, it would also relieve families of incredibly stressful experiences of the currently mandated food challenges in clinical trials."

"These changes," Dave said, "are quite feasible and will simply require productive meetings with all the constituents determined to safely bring therapies to market."

I couldn't agree more with the Bunnungs' thoughts. The trauma involved with feeding an allergic individual a food until they react to it, and then rushing to stop the reaction, is hard to overstate. Amazingly, these are the "entry criteria" for clinical trials for food allergy. The fact that food allergic individuals are willing to risk triggering a reaction to find treatment explains clearly the need for therapeutic relief and high lights the burden patients feel from avoidance. My hope and trust are in the future where we all—patients, scientists, doctors, pharmaceutical companies, public health groups, advocacy groups, farmers, the food manufacturing and restaurant industry, and the FDA—come together to bring an end to food allergies, which begs to be deemed a single disease like cancer despite different types. When you silo diseases, you risk losing sight on treatments and cures in one silo that can benefit another. The power of a collective, multidimensional force cannot be understated. The epidemic began in my lifetime and my dream is to see it pass in my lifetime.

To be sure, the exact cause of the allergy epidemic is currently unknown, but a few theories are being studied and debated by me and my colleagues that reflect both genetic and environmental forces that jointly act on an individual's immune system. Before we get to those theories, however, let's turn to the biology of a true food allergy and continue to sort through the complex maze of allergies and intolerances.

Fearless Facts

✦ Approximately thirty-two million Americans have food allergies, including six million children; that's 1 in 13 children and 1 in 10 adults. Nearly half of adults will develop at least one new food allergy after the age of eighteen.

✦ People can be allergic to any food, but the top nine food allergens are peanuts, milk, shellfish, tree nuts, eggs, finfish, wheat, soy, and sesame.

✦ One in 5 US adults reports that they may have a "food allergy," but about half of those folks may not have an allergy; rather, they suffer from another food-related condition, such as an intolerance.

→ Some of the most common intolerances are to dairy, gluten, caffeine, alcohol, MSG, salicylates, amines, FODMAPs, sulfites, fructose, and food dyes.

→ Across the wide spectrum of food allergy and intolerances, individuals can have a combination of both immunologic allergies and nonimmunologic conditions (a.k.a. "masqueraders"). Complicating this picture are autoimmune disorders such as celiac disease as well as gastrointestinal disorders, such as irritable bowel syndrome (IBS) and inflammatory bowel disease (IBD), which can also lead to similar food-induced symptoms.

two

"ALLERGIES" ARE NOT ALL CREATED EQUAL

Anatomy of Immune-Based Reactions vs. Masqueraders on the Spectrum

W HEN ROBERT GOT HIS FRIEND DAVE'S TEXT, HE REALIZED HE HAD NEVER actually taken a tally.

> **Text from Dave:** "Rob, how many allergic reactions have you had since college? I think we should have you make a video explaining food allergy doesn't end in childhood."
>
> **Text back from Rob**: "Probably 20–30."

That was just as an adult. Rob also had numerous anaphylactic reactions to peanuts as a child during a time in the 1970s when food allergy was a novel concept to most Americans. It was certainly unknown to him and his family until the summer of 1978, when he almost died. Rob had eaten peanut butter before, but never much cared for it. He chose to avoid peanuts and mostly did. But at a dimly lit cocktail party on a family cruise in the Arctic Sea, north of the North Cape of Norway, he ate a Thai satay—a beef skewer that he didn't realize was smothered in peanut sauce. He immediately felt ill and went to his cabin where he started to have trouble breathing. He looked at the mirror and could not recognize himself; his lips had swollen to the size of golf balls as his throat constricted. He called the ship's operator to have them find his parents and a doctor. Rob was eight years old.

Were it not for the Norwegian ship doctor who correctly diagnosed his ailment, administered epinephrine, and nursed Rob back to health, in his own estimation, he would be dead. And he would have been dead many times over throughout the next several decades as Rob learned to live with a potentially fatal peanut allergy. Now in his fifties, Rob sits on the National Board of Directors for FARE and enjoys a full life with his family and thriving business career in Los Angeles.

Alexi Ryann Stafford, fifteen, was not so fortunate. While at a friend's house on June 25, 2018, she took a cookie from an open package that had a red wrapping and looked similar to the type of cookies her parents had deemed safe for her. But the box actually contained a version of the cookies with peanut butter cups. She didn't see this fact because it was hidden by a pulled-back flap. Alexi had a severe peanut allergy. She only ate one cookie.

She immediately started feeling tingling in her mouth and went straight home. Her condition rapidly deteriorated. She went into ana-phylactic shock, stopped breathing, and became unconscious. Her parents administered two EpiPens while she was unconscious and waited for the paramedics to arrive. It felt like an eternity.

Alexi died within one and a half hours of eating that cookie.

Earlier that year, cashews took the life of thirty-one-year-old George Hodgkiss, who had survived two tours in both Iraq and Afghanistan. And in 2017, a Singapore woman, Ms. Khoo Siew Hong, was sixty years young when she made the fatal mistake of eating two prawns for lunch. She was allergic to shellfish, though she'd eaten prawns in the past without experiencing a reaction. A few hours later, paramedics were trying to resuscitate her; at the hospital, she was given twelve doses of epinephrine. She never regained consciousness and her family took her off the ventilator that night.

As you can tell from these stories, allergic reactions do not discriminate based on age, gender, or location. Although food allergies can be life-threatening, fatal reactions are rare. More common are severe reactions that send people to the ER and often require hospitalization. Fatal reactions claim about ten lives a year in the US, although it is difficult to truly estimate. Most times with the right medications and the body's own healing mechanisms, the majority recover. This is why it is so important to be able to get a diagnosis, recognize right away when a reaction commences, and treat it immediately, as even one life lost is one too many.

Every few minutes, someone seeks emergency help for scary biological responses to something they just ate. Sometimes they are first-time reactions to foods that were once harmless and enjoyed without a second thought. Other times, they occur in people who are accustomed to avoiding their food allergen, carefully read ingredient labels, and are prepared to treat themselves if they have an accidental reaction.

Because allergies are often thought of as a broad term encompassing many environmental, food, stinging insect, and medicine triggers, it is understandable why this confuses so many people. One may think of the stereotypical peanut or bee sting allergy or the adults who can't eat grains or have dairy. But it's much more complex than that. In this chapter I'm going to explain the biology of an allergic reaction in detail, including some less widely known reactions, such as pollen-food allergy syndrome (often related to fruits and vegetables), and the more recently defined alpha-gal allergy (related to mammalian meat consumption). These reactions take up a large portion of real estate on the spectrum of adverse food reactions.

We often think of sudden, catastrophic illness as a situation that strikes vulnerable people due to advanced age or a serious genetic anomaly. Stories of people who are otherwise superhealthy—they are young, fit, and strong—and who go from being fine to having trouble breathing and in an ambulance within minutes are exceptionally rare. But it can happen with food allergies. It's strange to consider, but everyday foods can cause serious reactions faster than any pathogenic virus or invasive bacteria.

ANATOMY OF AN ATTACK

Food allergies that incite the immune system produce symptoms that can affect the skin (e.g., hives, swelling, rash), gut (e.g., abdominal pain, vomiting, diarrhea), respiratory system (e.g., throat tightness, cough, trouble breathing, wheezing), and cardiovascular system (e.g., blood pressure drop, fainting). Anaphylaxis is the most severe reaction, which can be life-threatening when not promptly addressed. It is important to remind you—as I mentioned earlier—that the timing, sequence, and severity of symptoms can vary for the same individual, and previous reactions do not necessarily predict how severe future reactions will be. You might have hives and itching after eating a particular food one day, but then have anaphylaxis, including trouble breathing and drop in blood pressure, with the next exposure. Although it is not clear why some people are more likely to have a severe allergic reaction than others, this likely depends on an individual's sensitivity, the amount of food consumed, a concurrent viral illness, and other factors, such as strenuous activity around the time of allergen ingestion and having underlying uncontrolled asthma.

So, how does someone develop a life-threatening food allergy? First of all, the individual has to become *sensitized* to the food. This means that their immune system had some previous exposure to it, whether by eating it directly or having some contact with the potential allergen through the skin, which results in the development of allergic antibodies (IgE) and "sensitization."

Another important point is that we rarely develop a food allergy to something we consume regularly, because the body becomes used to the food—it's trained to know it's not an enemy to fight. In fact, these reasons are likely why the recent recommendations for early *oral* introduction and *regular* consumption of peanut to infants at high risk work and decrease the risk of developing peanut allergy by about 80 percent. (This could possibly be one puzzle piece in why many older children and adults become allergic to tree nuts and seafood—things they may not be consuming very regularly.)

At the heart of an immediate allergic reaction is immunoglobulin E (IgE), an antibody that's usually in low supply in the bloodstream but is the chief sentinel for allergens it encounters. And when it does find a potentially "harmful" substance in the body, it rapidly goes into overdrive and activates the release of other chemicals that can have enormous biological impact, causing symptoms most often in the nose, lungs, throat, sinuses, ears, lining of the stomach, or on the skin. One of the most talked-about chemicals unleashed in the chain of events is histamine, which causes tightening of the muscles in the airways and the dilation of blood vessels. Other chemicals are involved with other effects on tissues, but that's the overall picture from a very general standpoint. Now, let's slow down this conversation so you can grasp what takes place, one sequence at a time, on one extreme side of the spectrum.

Anaphylaxis in Slow Motion

It's important to understand that the immune system is a smart biological marvel, but it can become confused and misdirect its forces. Our immune system serves an important function: to protect us from infections and diseases. The human body is constantly under siege. It must defend itself from a whole host of bacterial, parasitic, and viral invaders, not to mention rogue cancerous cells. To put this into alarming perspective: Scientists at the University of British Columbia have estimated that 800 million viruses rain onto every square meter of the planet every day; at least 320,000 different viruses infect mammals; and at last count, there are 219 virus species that are known to be able to infect humans. The vast majority of viruses are harmless and, in some cases, can be beneficial to human health by, for instance, killing bad bacteria or fighting against more dangerous viruses. But as we all know from the experience with Covid-19 and horror stories about influenza, Ebola, HIV, and dengue fever, there are a few bad apples in the bunch that can inflict lots of harm.

The immune system has to distinguish between self (our normal cells), threats (infectious agents/abnormal cells), and harmless substances (foods, pollens, animal dander, etc.) that it should ignore. It should recognize and ignore our own chemical structure, known as "self antigens," while vigorously attacking foreign threats. The problem, however, is that it can label chemical structures, such as certain proteins in a cashew or crustacean, as a villain when it shouldn't. The immune system then tries to expel the "invader," and in doing so, wreaks havoc. It's as though the body declares war for no legitimate threat during times of peace.

The body craves what's called homeostasis—an equilibrium that keeps things physiologically balanced, steady, and harmonized (*homeostasis* is Greek for "same" and "steady"). The systems need to be maintained to be able to operate properly and deal with any challenges or perturbations. Classic examples include body temperature, blood sugar, calcium levels, and fluid volume, each of which strives to stay within normal, set limits. When certain conditions impact or threaten a body's homeostasis and, in turn, functionality, the body responds quickly to try to bring things under control again. It has built-in regulatory mechanisms that have evolved over millions of years to sustain our survival. Sweating, for example, cools the body when heat threatens its homeostatic temperature; blood pressure, blood sugar, and calcium levels are all kept in check, too, through rigorous homeostatic controls. But when there's confusion in the body's homeostatic controls, as in the case of misidentifying a food protein, the body can end up mistaking friend for foe—with disastrous results.

There are actually two types of reactions that can result in anaphylaxis: immunologic and nonimmunologic. Bear with me here because some of this language can come across as technical, but the concepts are important. The most common type of reaction is *immunologic*, which is when substances, such as pollen, certain foods, drugs, latex, mold, pet dander, dust mites, or insect stings, are recognized by the body as harmful allergens and trigger special immune cells called B cells to produce those IgE antibodies. This is what happens during allergic *sensitization*, which we just defined. These IgE molecules are Y-shaped proteins (globulins) that act like signal markers to seek out and find foreign material, such as those allergens. These antibodies travel to cells and dock themselves on the surface of mast cells and basophils (circulating white blood cells), which release mediators during allergic reactions. We use the term *mediators* in medicine to refer to key biochemical "signals" in the body, which are intermediary substances released from cells that regulate or cause physiologic consequences. Put another way, mast cells and basophils are like conductors of an orchestra that tell the immune system what to do when it encounters an allergen. Once activated, they release molecules that further communicate to other cells, chiefly white blood cells, and prime the immune system for action.

In addition to cytokines, which are the chemical signals, getting released, histamine floods the bloodstream (circulation). Histamine is a potent vasodilator—it immediately opens up blood vessels and, as a result, blood pools in the periphery instead of returning to the heart, pressure drops, and the entire circulatory system becomes compromised. This can impact the delivery of vital oxygen to tissues, including the heart and brain. At the same time, histamine can cause blood vessels to become leaky, allowing fluid to escape the vascular space, further lowering blood pressure and causing swelling throughout the body. As mentioned, other symptoms most often involve the nose, lungs, throat, sinuses, ears, lining of the stomach, or skin. IgE-specific antibodies for food allergens develop during initial sensitization to a food. Once sensitization occurs, food antigen–specific IgE is present in the circulation and on the surface of tissue mast cells and basophils. Those IgE soldiers are lying in wait and ready for a rapid, allergic response the next time an allergen it knows comes along. After reexposure to the food, the immune response causes a release of those myriad chemicals that foment a storm of sorts in the body, and that results in physical symptoms.

In the second type of anaphylaxis, often referred to as *anaphylactoid*, reactions are defined as those producing the same clinical picture with anaphylaxis but without the involvement of IgE. These anaphylactoid reactions either occur through a direct nonimmune-mediated release of substances from mast cells and basophils or result from what's called direct complement activation. Don't worry about what that means; just remember that anaphylactoid reactions involve a different biological pathway to the same symptoms and outcome (and they are also treated the same, with epinephrine). Histamines and cytokines are still released to do their thing to the circulatory system, but IgE is not a player. People can have nonimmunologic, anaphylactoid reactions to drugs, such as opioids (e.g., morphine, codeine), for example, in which the drug directly causes the release of those chemicals through the activation of the opioid receptor and without relying on IgE (as such, sometimes these reactions are called "pseudo-allergies").

Most people are familiar with how anaphylaxis affects one's breathing, which can become quickly labored or, in a worst-case scenario, impossible. How does this happen? In addition to histamine causing vasodilation, it triggers spasms of the bronchi, the main air passages to the lungs. These bronchospasms can make it difficult to breathe and might cause wheezing, similar to that during an asthma attack. Moreover, swelling in the throat can close off the airway, leading to further breathing difficulties. If you've ever taken a first-aid class, you may remember the importance of "ABC": compromised **A**irway, **B**reathing, and **C**irculation. A patient in this condition needs the airway to be opened, and blood pressure to be brought back up and maintained. These two actions help return circulation to normal.

The most important treatment of anaphylaxis is epinephrine, which helps open up the airways and constricts blood vessels. Antihistamines and intravenous (IV) fluids are important in restoring the person's healthy physiology during a severe anaphylactic attack. Remember earlier when we discussed how the release of histamine causes blood vessels to leak valuable fluid into the tissue (causing swelling)? Antihistamines and epinephrine can help stop that leakage, while IV fluids help fill those blood vessels back up and regain normal circulatory function.

Breathing difficulties can be divided into those affecting the upper and lower respiratory tract. Upper respiratory tract symptoms include common cold–like symptoms, such as sneezing, runny rose, congestion, nasal and/or eye itching, red eyes, and tearing. Lower respiratory signs and symptoms happen in up to 70 percent of anaphylactic reactions and include breathing difficulties, such as noisy breathing, chest tightness or pain, cough, wheezing, and a hoarse voice (you sound sick/muffled). (I should note that, medically speaking, sometimes the upper airway is thought of as being outside of the chest, so hoarseness and throat tightness could be considered symptoms of the upper airway.)

Gastrointestinal symptoms occur in 45 percent of cases of anaphylaxis. Many patients experience tingling or itching in their mouth. Young children may scratch at their mouth, tongue, throat, or ears. Nausea and vomiting can occur within minutes of ingestion, whereas abdominal pain, cramping, and diarrhea may occur either immediately or with a delay of up to several hours after ingestion. Vomiting in an IgE-mediated reaction also can happen within a couple of hours after ingestion. These symptoms can result in dehydration and electrolyte disturbances in infants and young children, and the general loss of fluids from the vomiting and diarrhea can result in what's called hypovolemic shock, a dangerous condition that makes it impossible for the heart to pump a sufficient amount of blood to the body (this can also happen in food protein–induced enterocolitis syndrome [FPIES] reactions).

Cardiovascular symptoms also can occur in 45 percent of cases of anaphylaxis, which makes sense given the downstream effects from the changes to the circulatory system I've already described in response to those biochemicals flooding the system. Worse-case scenarios include loss of blood pressure so severe that cardiac arrest can result—although

I should temper this with a note that such reactions are not common, especially if medical help is present.

Most anaphylactic symptoms can occur within minutes after a reaction. However, *biphasic anaphylaxis* is the reoccurrence of these same symptoms hours after the initial reaction. This is also known as a *biphasic reaction*. Think of this as a second reaction that occurs with no additional food exposure. This second reaction can be variable and just as severe as the initial anaphylactic event and can involve similar symptoms. In a recent study we published, 16.4 percent of people with food allergy reported a biphasic reaction, about 1 in 10 children and 1 in 5 adults. The time interval between biphasic reactions can range from several hours to one to two days, but most secondary reactions occur within eight hours of the initial reaction. For this reason, it's important to continue monitoring yourself or your loved one for any late-occurring food-allergic reactions. Appropriate treatment may include additional epinephrine injections. This is why allergists recommend having at least two epinephrine autoinjectors on hand at all times. It's critical to recognize biphasic reactions so that you are prepared to treat and seek additional medical care as indicated.

Although anaphylaxis only affects a small percentage of the general population, food allergies are the most common cause of anaphylaxis at all ages outside a hospital. We found over 40 percent of children with food allergy had experienced a severe allergic reaction and 1 in 5 children went to the emergency department for an allergic reaction in the past year. Given the troubling rise in food allergies, these numbers may increase if we don't do something about it. It is important to note that any food allergy can cause anaphylaxis, although in children, we mostly hear about peanut, and in adults, shellfish. The biggest risk factors for food-induced anaphylaxis are adolescent or young adult age, underlying uncontrolled asthma, and previous episodes of anaphylaxis. Overall, 15 percent of people who experience anaphylaxis also show neurological symptoms, often characterized "feelings of impending doom," headache, or confusion. Young children and infants can suddenly have unexplained behavioral changes, such as being irritable, clingy, and not wanting to play. This is when it's key to recognize those symptoms and respond accordingly.

The risk for anaphylaxis has classically been attributed to the nine foods listed on page 7, some medications, insect venom, and latex. But more recently, scientists have documented reactions from other sources or settings that further add more intriguing, albeit perplexing, color to the tapestry that's food allergy. Let's go there next.

Alpha-Gal Syndrome

Can an avid, lifelong meat-eater suddenly become allergic to a juicy steak? You bet. The only known IgE-mediated food allergy that characteristically has a delayed reaction is allergy to a sugar molecule called galactose-alpha-1,3-galactose (simplified to "alpha-gal"). This is an allergic reaction to a carbohydrate molecule on beef, pork, and lamb (nonprimate mammalian meats). Additional mammalian meats include bison, venison, goat, horse, rabbit, squirrel, kangaroo, antelope, buffalo, camel, guinea pig, bat, and whale. In contrast to the immediate allergic reactions that occur after eating such foods as peanut, egg, and shellfish, an alpha-gal reaction is not typically apparent until four to six hours after meat ingestion. Symptoms are similar to other IgE-mediated food allergies, with hives, severe itching, and gastrointestinal symptoms being most prevalent. And some people do progress down the path to full anaphylactic shock as described earlier, with serious cardiovascular and respiratory issues.

For most people with alpha-gal allergy or syndrome, avoiding those problematic meats is enough to prevent further reactions. But some people continue to have reactions and require additional elimination of dairy and gelatin to fully avoid reactions, because alpha-gal is also found in primarily cow's, sheep's, and goat's milk as well as bovine gelatin. Although you may think gelatin is a very specific and easy-to-recognize ingredient, this protein product made from animal tissue (mostly collagen) is used as a stabilizer, thickener, texturizer, fat replacement, and binding agent in a wide variety of foods, including candies and drinks (those marshmallow confections, for example, that you find around Easter and Halloween contain gelatin; it's what makes them squishy). It's also used in some pharmaceuticals, such as gummy vitamins, and vaccines, such as flu shots. Gelatin is commonly derived from cows and pigs, but can also come from chickens and fish. Gelatin allergy itself is rare but should be ruled out to prevent future reactions. For those with alpha-gal syndrome, avoiding all forms of gelatin is safest.

Where the alpha-gal story really gets interesting is in its origin: the Lone Star tick's saliva. You read that right: certain species of ticks deliver the sugar molecule through their bite and in susceptible people, their immune system reacts—setting the body up for a lifelong allergy to red meat (e.g., beef, pork, lamb, and other mammalian products). My colleague Dr. Thomas Platts-Mills was the first to discover this linkage between alpha-gal allergy and Lone Star tick bites in 2002.

The Lone Star tick, along with other ticks, are found predominantly in the southeastern United States, and most cases of alpha-gal syndrome occur in this region. But the condition appears to be spreading farther north and west as deer carry the Lone Star tick to new parts of the United States and the general tick populations grow and expand into new regions. Alpha-gal syndrome also has been diagnosed in Europe, Australia, Asia, and South Africa, where other types of ticks carry alpha-gal molecules.

Scientifically, we don't fully understand this newly emerging allergy, and what's particularly fascinating about it is that the reaction is delayed by several hours, unlike other typical food allergies. So, it's not uncommon for someone with alpha-gal allergy to eat a steak for dinner, go to bed feeling fine, and then wake up in the middle of the night to such reaction symptoms as hives, swelling, wheezing, and/or abdominal pain. These delayed reactions are likely related to the time it takes for the antigen (the alpha-gal molecule) to be digested and/or processed, so the allergic form of the sugar molecule doesn't enter the circulation until several hours after eating. And, as you can imagine, when you wake up with the reaction, your mind is probably not going to think back directly to the steak.

Alpha-gal is the only known carbohydrate antigen to induce an IgE-mediated reaction, as all the remainder are due to proteins. When people who live where these ticks are common and they have a delayed reaction to red meat or recurrent skin rashes and swelling, and unexplained anaphylaxis, alpha-gal allergy might be the culprit. Interestingly, when scientists were trying to establish the alpha-gal mystery in the early to mid-2000s and tease out its origins, they found themselves connecting some intriguing dots: the geographical distribution of the meat reactions were happening primarily in the same regions—chiefly in a group of southern US states—where people experienced reactions to cetuximab, which is a chemotherapy drug used to treat metastatic colorectal cancer, metastatic non-small cell lung cancer, and head and neck cancer. The anti-cancer medication (brand name Erbitux) also contains alpha-gal. People who have allergic reactions to this drug have a higher risk for red meat allergy and are likely to have been bitten by ticks in the past. In these vulnerable cancer patients, their reactions to cetuximab are often immediate because the drug is delivered intravenously.

We now think that when people have frequent, unexplained anaphylactic reactions yet who test negative for other food allergies, alpha-gal syndrome could be the culprit for which the only treatment is avoidance of red meat products. The time-delayed reaction of alpha-gal syndrome is thought to be due to the alpha-gal molecules taking longer than other allergens to be digested and enter the circulatory system. More research is needed to understand the connection between ticks that carry alpha-gal in certain regions and cases of alpha-gal syndrome that don't seem directly linked to tick bites.

Food-Dependent Exercise-Induced Anaphylaxis

This allergy is a wild one because it seemingly gives people a reason to say they are "allergic" to exercise. Food-dependent exercise-induced anaphylaxis is when people physically exert themselves within a few hours of eating and then experience symptoms of anaphylaxis. This can also be very challenging for active people or athletes with allergies or going through oral immunotherapy (Chapter 7). I know a very active young adult who had a hard time not eating and not exercising and would have periodic reactions, some causing anaphylaxis requiring epinephrine.

Symptoms typically begin during vigorous exercise, but the level of exertion that precipitates symptoms is unpredictable. Interestingly, these people do not have reactions if they consume the foods to which they are sensitized without exercising afterward. And although most individuals with this experience only have symptoms to specific foods to which they are sensitized, some patients can experience anaphylaxis if they exercise after consuming *any* food or drink (hence the "allergy to exercise"). The most common food triggers are wheat, dairy, and shellfish, but other triggers of this unusual reaction include some fruits and vegetables, aspirin, anti-inflammatories (NSAIDS), alcohol, extreme temperatures, humidity, and even hormonal changes.

Like alpha-gal allergy, we don't fully understand this type of allergy, other than it follows the same biology as traditional allergies with the usual players, such as IgE, mast cells, and histamine release, but we don't know how exercise specifically triggers the cascade of events. A number of hypotheses are currently being studied, including how exercise changes one's physiology in the context of having ingested certain foods. Much more is to be learned about this allergy, a rare and underdiagnosed one. It was first described in 1979 as a case report of shellfish allergy that only manifested itself in the presence of exercise. But today, the most common culprits when combined with exercise are wheat

(80 percent), alcohol (25 percent), nonsteroidal anti-inflammatories such as ibuprofen (9 percent), and heat (5 percent). It can start at any age, but typically strikes people at the ages they are most physically active—between four and seventy-four years old. I've heard of cases where doctors trying to diagnose this allergy have their patients eat the potentially offending food with red wine and then run up and down the road until symptoms develop!

People with this unusual disorder must carefully control their triggers in combination with their exercise habits. It is an individualized approach as some may completely avoid the food and others just around the time of exercise. Later on, we'll see how exercise can also factor into oral immunotherapy (OIT), a treatment option for food allergy, as some people are more prone to an adverse reaction during OIT if they exert physical effort. Exercise around the time of dosing increases the chance of a reaction so timing of both the dosing and exercise becomes important.

POLLEN-FOOD ALLERGY SYNDROME (PFAS)/
ORAL ALLERGY SYNDROME (OAS)

This is one of the most common masqueraders. This is also one that is important to get right, as you may not need to avoid the culprit food all the time. There's a lot of confusion over the distinction between "classic" food allergy to fruits and vegetables and *pollen-food allergy syndrome* (PFAS, a.k.a. oral allergy syndrome [OAS]); we'll stick with PFAS in terminology going forward, as it's the more accepted language today. Both PFAS and classic food allergy to fruits and vegetables involve rapid allergic reactions occurring immediately after eating particular raw fruits (e.g., apples, peaches, cherries) or vegetables (e.g., carrots, celery), and some tree nuts, peanuts, and seeds. Individuals with PFAS react to the food because they are allergic to pollens (e.g., from birch, mugwort, ragweed, grass) whose molecular structure is similar enough to the raw food proteins that their immune system "mistakes" the food for a pollen. In other words, the body confuses a fruit protein with a pollen protein, and IgE antibodies that were created in response to pollen instead produce an allergic reaction to fruit. When this happens, the person usually has a mild skin reaction or itchy mouth/throat when they touch or eat the raw fruit or vegetable. Because the potential culprits to PFAS can involve foods that cause a serious allergic reaction in people, such as almonds, soybeans, walnuts, hazelnuts, peanuts, and sunflower seeds, deciphering between food allergy and PFAS on the spectrum can be tricky. It requires careful attention to the symptoms and testing that can determine cross reactivity to pollen allergens.

The symptoms of PFAS include itchy mouth, scratchy throat, or swelling of the lips, mouth, tongue, and throat; itchy ears and hives on the mouth are sometimes reported (only 3 percent will have such symptoms as tightness in the throat, difficulty swallowing, and nausea). The symptoms rarely progress beyond the mouth and throat, but a full-on anaphylactic response is possible (in less than 2 percent of people with PFAS), especially if someone drinks the uncooked fruits/vegetables quickly, such as in a smoothie. However, most people affected by PFAS can usually eat the same fruits or vegetables in cooked or pickled form because the proteins are distorted (denatured) during the heating process, and the immune system no longer recognizes the food.

Pollen-food allergy syndrome typically does not appear in young children, but it can in some cases. It arrives in older children, teens, and young adults who have been eating the fruits or vegetables in question for years without any problems. I remember one of my pediatric residents who thought she had a food allergy to tomatoes, and after talking with her, we figured out she had PFAS. She was so excited to understand her diagnosis and actually went on to become a practicing allergist. Young children under the age of three do not usually develop allergic rhinitis (hay fever) until after they are toddlers, but some are sensitized by one year of age and can show signs of seasonal symptoms as early as eighteen months. Hay fever is associated with reactions to the pollens that cross-react with the foods. PFAS is highly variable and people with PFAS may react to one food or many foods; we don't understand what determines the extent of PFAS. Although not everyone with a pollen allergy experiences PFAS when eating the following foods, they are commonly associated with these allergens (for a more comprehensive list, see the chart on pages 40–41):

→ Birch tree pollen: apple, almond, carrot, celery, cherry, hazelnut, kiwifruit, peach, peanut, pear, plum
→ Grass pollen: celery, melon, orange, peach, tomato
→ Ragweed pollen: banana, cucumber, melon, sunflower seeds, zucchini
→ Mugwort: bell pepper, broccoli, cabbage, cauliflower, fennel, onion

Cross-reactivities—being allergic to one particular substance while also reacting to related substances, as in the case of the fruit-pollen phenomenon—can happen with other triggers. Cross-reactivities can be common, for instance, between different species of fish, tree nuts or seeds, cow's milk and milk from other mammals (e.g., goat's or sheep's milk), and the most unusual one of all: a relationship between being allergic to latex—the natural rubber that comes from a plant and is found in many products we come into contact with—and certain fruits, such as avocado, banana, chestnut, papaya, and kiwifruit. This association between latex sensitivity and food allergy is often referred to as the latex-fruit syndrome. But again, these types of reactions are usually mild, confined to one area of the body, such as the mouth or skin, and usually do not elicit anaphylaxis.

Pollen-Food Allergy Syndrome
(PFAS, or Oral Allergy Syndrome)

Season	SPRING	SUMMER	LATE SUMMER–FALL	FALL
Pollen implicated in the oral cross-reactivity reactions with foods	Birch	Timothy and orchard grass	Ragweed	Mugwort
FRUIT				
Pitted Fruit				
Apple	X			
Apricot	X			
Cherry	X			
Peach	X	X		
Pear	X			
Plum	X			
Melons				
Cantaloupe			X	
Honeydew			X	
Watermelon		X	X	
Other				
Banana			X	
Kiwifruit	X			
Orange		X		
Strawberry	X			
Tomato		X		
VEGETABLES				
Bell pepper				X
Broccoli				X
Cabbage				X

Season	SPRING	SUMMER	LATE SUMMER-FALL	FALL
VEGETABLES (continued)				
Carrot	X			
Cauliflower				X
Celery	X			
Chard				X
Cucumber			X	
Garlic				X
Onion				X
Parsley	X			X
White potato		X	X	
Zucchini			X	
SPICES				
Aniseed				X
Black pepper				X
Caraway				X
Coriander				X
Fennel				X
LEGUMES*				
Peanut	X			
Soybean	X			
NUTS*				
Almond	X			
Hazelnut	X			

*Mouth or throat itching from peanut, soybean, almond, and hazelnut could signal the first signs of a more serious food issue with the potential for anaphylaxis. See an allergist/immunologist if such symptoms are noted.

This chart was adapted from the American Academy of Allergy, Asthma, and Immunology. For more information, go to www.aaaai.org.

Eosinophilic Esophagitis (EoE) and
Eosinophilic Gastrointestinal Disorders (EGID)

In the first chapter, I briefly defined eosinophilic esophagitis (EoE), a chronic, allergic inflammatory disease of the esophagus. It occurs when a type of white blood cell, the eosinophil, accumulates in the esophagus and causes injury and inflammation and is a type of an eosinophilic gastrointestinal disorder (EGID). EGID can occur in the esophagus, stomach, and colon with an increased number of eosinophils in the gastrointestinal system causing inflammation. The symptoms of EGID are nausea, vomiting, abdominal pain, and occasionally diarrhea—symptoms that can appear to be signs of other GI conditions, such as irritable bowel syndrome (IBS) or inflammatory bowel disease (IBD), an umbrella term that, as previously defined, includes Crohn's disease and ulcerative colitis.

Our team recently surveyed over fifty thousand US households and concluded that approximately 1 in 600 Americans have been diagnosed with EoE, with similar rates seen among children and adults. Remarkably, among these people with EoE, 1 in 3 has a food allergy. Rates of other allergic conditions (e.g., asthma, eczema, allergic rhinitis) were also much higher among those individuals with EoE, suggesting that EoE may be a later step along the "allergic march" that emerges alongside or following the development of food allergy. Allergists like to think of EoE as a chronic inflammatory disease of the esophagus that often involves food allergies, but not always.

Symptoms of EoE in children may include poor weight gain, difficulty feeding, vomiting, food refusal, feeding intolerance, chest pain, abdominal pain, and difficulty swallowing with food impaction. I like to refer to EoE as atopic dermatitis of the gastrointestinal tract. Many children I know were first diagnosed with food allergies, and as time went on, it was discovered they had EoE as well. In fact, this happened with two of my very close friends. Their children both had food allergies, and slowly they recognized symptoms of difficulty swallowing and coughing and also noticed poor growth. In one case after diagnosis, a gastrostomy tube (G-tube) needed to be placed to provide adequate nutrition while determining the exact food culprits. Although rare, in some cases children end up getting a G-tube for a period of time to help with nutrition and growth. A G-tube is a tube inserted through the belly that brings nutrition directly to the stomach, skipping the esophagus. Identifying EoE early and getting care from a knowledgeable gastroenterologist, allergist, and dietitian team is essential. Again, due to the overlapping symptoms EoE shares with other esophageal and gastrointestinal disorders, diagnosing EoE can be delayed in a primary care setting. But more and more, physicians are becoming increasingly aware of this unique condition and can tease it apart from the many other potential diagnoses that involve the digestive system.

Eosinophilic esophagitis is a chronic immune system disease on the food reaction spectrum. It was first reported in 1978 but has only been identified more widely in the past two decades and is now considered a major cause of digestive system (gastrointestinal) illness. (Only since 2007 has EoE been recognized as a distinct new condition.) Allergists and gastroenterologists are seeing many more patients with EoE, and though it's not always outgrown, it can be medically managed. (Originally, eosinophilic esophagitis was thought to be a childhood disease, but now it is known to be common in adults as well.) A doctor's first order of business, however, is ruling out other causes of the symptoms that mimic EoE, such as gastroesophageal reflux disease (GERD), physical obstructions in the esophagus, such as a cancerous malignancy, and others.

While the exact cause of EoE is not yet known, the general belief is that it's typically caused by an immune response to specific foods and it has both underlying genetic and environmental forces at work. Many patients with EoE have food allergies or other allergic diseases, such as hay fever, asthma, and/or eczema; researchers have identified a number of genes that play a role in developing EoE. It appears to run in families, hence a genetic component. Environment matters, too, as people who live in a cold or dry climate are more likely to be diagnosed with eosinophilic esophagitis than those in other climates. Not surprisingly, an individual is more likely to be diagnosed between the spring and fall, probably because levels of pollen and other allergens are higher and people are more likely to be outdoors.

Unfortunately, the only way to currently diagnose EoE is through biopsies taken from the esophagus via endoscopy and counting the number of eosinophils that are present in the tissue. Thankfully, new and less invasive diagnostics are on the horizon. Patients often benefit from seeing a team of people at a multidisciplinary center that enlists the experience of GI doctors, allergists, dietitians, feeding specialists, and often a social worker and a psychologist. The advantage is that patients can see multiple providers on the same day to discuss the situation and design an individualized plan going forward.

We still have a lot to learn about EoE and treatment for it; many researchers all over the world are on it. Currently, one treatment for both children and adults includes eliminating the top allergens from the diet and then possibly adding one at a time back in and checking with endoscopy (using a long, thin camera) whether it is okay. However, this is quite cumbersome and tedious for patients and their families. Thankfully, new advances in better diagnostics that can detect the inflammation without needing the sedation and endoscopy are under development alongside potential new treatments. Other common treatments include ingested topical steroids. I have families doing both and sometimes switching between these approaches.

My colleague and dear friend Dr. Anna Nowak-Wegrzyn is director of the Pediatric Allergy Program at Hassenfeld Children's Hospital at NYU Langone in New York Health. Like me, she works with children and their parents to treat allergies and to prevent new allergies from developing in the future. She also happens to specialize in EoE. "It's a long-term inflammatory condition that has its good days and bad days, though it can go into remission," she says. "Patients tend to be very overall allergic, and when the pollen counts are high, their EoE symptoms worsen. For reasons we don't know, there's a higher prevalence among males than females."

In addition to controlling environmental triggers, such as exposure to pollen, to be able to help manage the condition, it is important to discuss management strategies with your allergist and gastroenterologist through shared decision, as there are a couple of options depending on what is best for you and your family. Patients can eliminate common foods (milk, wheat, egg, soy, nuts, seafood) that trigger EoE from their diet or be managed with inhaled corticosteroid or a liquid solution steroid called viscous budesonide without any changes to the diet.

In infants and older children whose EoE does not resolve with these treatments, an elemental diet—specially formulated liquid preparations—is more than 90 percent effective in relieving active inflammation. Elemental diets provide supplemental nutrition with special amino acid–based formulas; these formulas do not elicit an allergic response and can help patients safely fulfill their nutritional needs. A number of biologics are also under development for EoE (more on biologics in Chapter 7).

Although EoE itself will not cause anaphylaxis, people who suffer from EoE occasionally have the kinds of food allergies that can land one in the emergency room from possible food impaction due to the inflamed esophagus. So, comprehensive management is key to controlling esophageal inflammation. As to why the emergence of EoE is on this expansive and increasingly complicated spectrum? Well, to answer that we need to turn to why there is a rise in food allergies in general.

Fearless Facts

→ Food allergies that incite the immune system—far left side of the spectrum—produce symptoms that can affect the skin (e.g., hives, swelling, rash), gut (e.g., abdominal pain, vomiting, diarrhea), respiratory system (e.g., throat tightness, cough, trouble breathing, wheezing), and cardiovascular system (e.g., blood pressure drop, fainting).

→ Anaphylaxis is the most severe allergic reaction, which can be life-threatening when not promptly addressed.

→ At the center of an immediate allergic reaction is immunoglobulin E (IgE), an antibody that rapidly goes into overdrive and activates the release of other chemicals that can have enormous biological impact.

→ In addition to the top nine food allergens, other immune-based reactions include alpha-gal allergy or syndrome (to meat), food-dependent exercise-induced anaphylaxis (to certain foods followed by exercise), eosinophilic gastrointestinal disorders (to substances that cause a built-up of specialized white blood cells and inflammation in the gastrointestinal tract), and pollen-food allergy syndrome/oral allergy syndrome (to certain fruits and vegetables). These other reactions are important to diagnose so you know how to manage them when they occur.

three

THE GENOME, EPIGENOME, MICROBIOME, AND RISK FOR ALLERGIES

Why Our Body Can Become Confused, Bewildered, and Inflamed

GIDEON LACK IS A PROFESSOR OF PEDIATRIC ALLERGY AT KING'S COLLEGE London who has a long and storied history in the field. More than twenty years ago, he met his match in his scientific endeavors when he encountered a mystifying contradiction to solve. As he is an internationally recognized authority on food allergies, you may be familiar with his research findings showing the benefits of feeding peanut products during infancy, which have led to a paradigm shift in food allergy prevention.

In 1998, Lack introduced his Dual Allergen Exposure Hypothesis in the pages of the *Lancet*. According to this revolutionary—paradoxical— theory, the development of allergies can occur as a result of two powerful circumstances: (1) compromised skin in a baby, due to such conditions as eczema, who is then exposed topically from protein residues in the home, on family members, or on surfaces that penetrate the skin and set up an abnormal immune response; and (2) delayed oral exposure to food proteins, such as peanuts, that prevent the body from establishing a normal tolerance to those proteins. In other words, babies who are not given peanuts (or peanut-containing foods) when they start eating solid foods at around four to six months of age are *more likely* to develop an allergy to peanuts than are babies who begin to consume peanut-based ingredients in their meals. Which is to say: we can potentially decrease the risk of developing food allergies by ensuring a baby's skin is healthy, and feed potential food allergens, such as peanuts, early in life. The thinking used to be that withholding introduction to peanut-containing foods for at least a year (sometimes longer) could protect infants from these potentially harmful proteins. But now that thinking has been totally reversed, based on dramatic new evidence. We now know that the longer you wait to feed an infant certain allergenic foods, the greater their potential risk of developing allergies to those foods.

In 2000, guidelines released by the American Academy of Pediatrics (AAP) recommended not to start peanut products in babies at high risk for developing food allergies mainly based on family history before their third birthday. This may have come in response to the rise in peanut allergy and fear around unknown causes for this rise. But that didn't help, and incidence of food allergies continued to climb. By 2008, with no data supporting the effectiveness of delayed allergen introduction, the AAP overturned their previous recommendation and let pediatricians and parents decide. And in 2017, the National Institute of Allergy and Infectious Diseases (NIAID) published new recommendations for preventing peanut allergy in all babies especially those at high risk due to their eczema. These guidelines were based on an expert panel review that I was fortunate to be a part of, looking at all of the current evidence from clinical studies, including the landmark study by Lack's group called LEAP (Learning Early About Peanut Allergy). Most notably, the new guidelines recommend introducing a baby to peanut-containing foods as early as four to six months of age, to help reduce their risk of developing food allergies. The new guidelines recommend early introduction of peanut-containing foods as early as four months of age for high-risk infants with severe eczema and around six months for low-risk infants. Other food items should be introduced to the infants first, and a common way to do this is by mixing 2 teaspoons of smooth peanut butter with about 2 teaspoons of water. (More information on this is in Appendix A.) Introducing allergens like peanut products to babies at high risk for peanut allergy, starting as early as 4–6 months, may help reduce the risk of developing peanut allergies by up to 80 percent.

As can happen in medicine, it often takes the chance convergence of many repeated observations made by a scientist with experience over time, as well as the dismissal of some ingrained dogma coupled with some ingenuity and intuition, to propose a new theory. "We've known about tolerance in medical literature for decades, but never applied it to humans," Lack says. Decades ago when he was working in Denver, Colorado, training as a postdoctoral allergy fellow, he was trying to make mice allergic to the egg protein albumin while studying asthma in a mouse model. Much to his chagrin, he discovered that if he fed young mice albumin, it was impossible to make them allergic. Albumin is well-known adjuvant to IgE, meaning it helps stir the pot in the animals' immune system to make them allergic. Adjuvants in medicine are substances that enhance the body's immune response to an antigen. But his mentor, Dr. Erwin Gelfand, said if he fed baby mice or rats a food protein, they will never become allergic to that food. That was a huge clue that would later pave the way for his monumental findings. A German colleague was simultaneously working on a model for eczema. His colleague noted that if he slightly abraded the mice's skin and put low doses of albumin in their skin, they eventually had an allergic response. "I didn't put the two and two together for a long time," Dr. Lack laments. Flash-forward a decade when Lack is back in the UK and seeing a lot of babies with peanut allergies whose mothers had followed all the guidelines. Avoidance wasn't working.

Around this time, Lack noticed something interesting: Peanut allergy in Jewish children living in the UK was about ten times more common than it was in Jewish children living in Israel. Since these children shared a similar ancestry (i.e., genetic background), the difference had to be something they were being exposed to in their environment. It turned out there was a big dietary difference. Children in the UK rarely ate peanut products in the first year or so of life—whereas infants in Israel commonly ate Bamba, a corn puff made with peanut butter, as a teething snack. He wondered: Could this be the important difference—that the Israeli children ate peanut products from an early age? Was Bamba acting as an inoculate of sorts against food allergy, in this case peanut allergy?

So, he and his colleague Dr. George du Toit, to name a few of the many who contributed, decided to test their hypothesis in an effort that would become the famous LEAP study published in the *New England Journal of Medicine* in 2015. Lack and his team recruited 640 babies who had severe eczema or egg allergy, which are known to increase the risk of subsequent development of peanut allergies. They divided them up into two groups: one was given Bamba to eat regularly (if they didn't like Bamba, they could eat smooth peanut butter), and the other was kept away from foods containing peanuts. They did this until the children were five years old.

At five years, only 3 percent of the kids who ate peanut products were allergic to peanuts—compared with 17 percent of those who didn't eat peanuts. This included infants whose immune systems were already producing IgE antibodies to peanut protein—that is to say, they were "sensitized" to peanut. Notably, those patients with strong positive tests were not included in the study due to safety concerns. When this landmark research study was published, I along with a group of national experts worked with the NIAID to develop new guidelines in 2017 that could help pediatricians and parents interpret and apply these findings toward the prevention of peanut allergy. The AAP endorsed the guidelines in 2019, and in an updated report, highlight their importance. An important note in this is that some infants at highest risk with severe eczema may have already developed peanut allergy, so it is important, if your baby is at high risk, to discuss this with your pediatrician and get to an allergist for evaluation as early as possible at around four months of age.

In hindsight, Lack has some intriguing insights all of us in the scientific community would do well to consider: "We design studies based on conceptual confusion. The cause of the disease is not the same as a trigger of a disease. Or as we say in more technical terms: Cause is pathogenesis; trigger is different. An example might help: if you die of a heart attack, the trigger could have been a blocked artery cutting off vital blood to the organ; but the underlying cause could have been coronary artery disease from living a long time with such risk factors as smoking, diabetes, and high blood pressure.

"For years we thought the cause and the trigger were one and the same. When you take a five-year-old with a peanut allergy and give her peanuts, she will have a reaction. We assumed that eating food was the trigger of the reaction, so the logic then says avoid that food to prevent development of the disease. That's conflating two different issues. One is the cause and one is the trigger."

He offers a fitting analogy to drive this point home: people with heart disease, such as angina, used to be told to avoid exercise, under the thinking that physical activity would trigger a cardiac event. Today, the advice is exactly the opposite: exercise can help prevent the progression of the heart disease. It's protective much in the way early introduction to allergenic foods are. Now, my colleagues and I like to share the following motto: *Through the skin, allergies could begin. Through the diet, allergies can stay quiet.*

The message is simple: prevent and treat eczema so babies' skin remains as healthy and intact as possible so allergens cannot penetrate, and begin to introduce babies at four to six months of age, when they are developmentally ready to eat a diverse array of foods. As a pediatrician researching the world of food allergies with a daughter who avoided peanuts and had severe eczema as an infant, I feel I have found my calling. My goal is to find answers to the potentially avoidable triggers to the development of food allergies.

Based on my experience and research, which I'll detail in Appendix A, my personal recommendation is to introduce one new food every one to two days and start diversifying the diet and enjoying the process with your baby. We'll be revisiting these key concepts later on, as well as think about the following: Are we medicalizing food introduction too much in infants? After all, around many parts of the world, infants eat what parents are eating, chewed up or watered down a bit.

It's an intriguing question, one that dovetails with other pieces to the puzzle of modern food allergies. When you think about how mothers fed their babies hundreds to thousands of years ago (clearly, before the invention of food manufacturing, utensils, and the whole concept of "baby food" or formula), a mother would prechew the food for her baby and use her bare hands to deliver it. Those hands, mind you, were far from sterile; the mother would have touched many things in her natural environment, in the process exposing her child's developing immune system to a diverse assortment of microbes.

While that is not how we live or wish to live today, that scenario provides a healthy immune challenge for the baby. As my colleague, Dr. Scott Sicherer, puts it, who is chief of the Division of Allergy and Immunology in the Department of Pediatrics and Director of the Jaffe Food Allergy Institute at Icahn School of Medicine at Mount Sinai: "Normal feeding practices before companies made baby foods and we became industrialized involved mouth to hand to mouth or mouth to mouth feeding of babies, otherwise they would have choked! Premastication is still evident in various cultures. It meant a diverse diet representing what the community was eating, given with plenty of communal germs! I also proposed that kissing is a vestige of this natural tendency, love is mouth to mouth feeding." Again, we'll explore these fascinating pieces of information later. For now, let's turn to the broader question of why food allergies in general are on the rise—not just peanut allergy and not just in children.

NOT JUST PEANUTS AND NOT JUST KIDS ANYMORE

Eczema has been identified as a top risk factor for the development of peanut allergy and probably most other allergies. I know this well as my daughter had severe eczema as an infant and went on to develop peanut, egg, and tree nut allergies. At that time, we did not know what we know now and the recommendation was to avoid peanuts. I should add that the rise in eczema is not without its own causes. Although genetics play into the development of eczema, there are other factors contributing to its severity and to the food allergy epidemic: cleanliness, especially when we look at how sterilized our lifestyle had become in comparison to previous generations, and yet we have the same immune system that demands to be challenged during its healthy development. We often bathe daily, using powerful (sometimes antimicrobial) chemical compounds that have only emerged within the past fifty to seventy years—a blink of the eye in evolutionary terms. Many babies are excessively bathed and certain products we use on their skin could be compromising their skin's barrier.

Don't get me wrong: bathing is important to hygiene at every age from zero to one hundred, and once eczema is present, daily bathing done right is very important. But bathing can transform from a healthy behavior to an unhealthy risk factor if you use the wrong products and/ or too harshly scrub the skin. Normal skin should be slightly acidic, but we tend to use lots of creams and lotions that are alkaline and which can strip the skin of natural oils and even damage the skin's natural microbiome—the protective microbes that live on the skin and contribute to its barrier function. Add to that the skin brushes and loofahs we use and it's easy to see how the process can quickly turn abrasive. (Ask any dermatologist about the epidemic of other skin conditions, including adult acne, and they will tell you: when we overwash and overscrub, we set the stage for problems.) I'll be going into much more detail later on these matters, but I bring them up now so you can begin to grasp the complexity of this topic.

The range of potential allergenic foods is just as wide and diverse as the food reaction spectrum itself. Although we have nine top or common allergens, more than 170 foods have been reported by the National Institute of Allergy and Infectious Diseases to cause bona fide allergic reactions. And virtually any food can trigger an intolerance to it at any age. The question we have to be asking is *Why?* What is causing this disquieting trend? What has changed to confuse our body? Let's delve deeper and explore what we in fact do know from high-profile research and what still needs to be figured out. The science tells us that the plausible answer is a combination of genetic and environmental factors and how they impact our biology. We'll start with a clear understanding of true food allergies as I defined them in the previous chapter.

WIRED FOR ALLERGIES

Can you be predisposed to having food allergies due to your genetic makeup? You bet. Having a parent or sibling with a food allergy increases your propensity. Scientists continue to identify genetic contributors to certain allergies. We know, for example, that a gene called c11orf30/ EMSY (EMSY for short) is associated with food allergy (which means EMSY could be a useful target for predicting and managing food allergy treatments in the future). Individuals with a certain mutation in the so-called filaggrin gene also have been found to be at increased risk for eczema, which you know now is a major risk factor for developing food allergies (much more on this in Chapter 8). This gene has an important barrier function in the epidermis or upper layer of the skin.

At the Sean N. Parker Center for Allergy and Asthma Research, led by my colleague Kari Nadeau, MD, PhD, and where I serve as a scientific executive committee member, they have further found that increased exposure to environmental pollutants, such as cigarette smoke and car exhaust, leads to the formation of chemical tags (what are called "epigenetic modifications") on the DNA of a key gene, Foxp3, involved in asthma—another risk factor for setting food allergies in motion. This likely helps explain why inhabitants of communities with high levels of air pollution are at a greater risk for developing both asthma and food allergies.

To be sure, epigenetic modifications, which act as On and Off switches to the genetic code, regulate the expression of genes and may contribute to the rapid rise in asthma and allergic diseases. Our genes may be relatively static, but changes in our surrounding environment can affect the way that these genes express themselves, leading the same DNA to behave differently when certain environmental influences are present. The International Society for Developmental Origins of Health and Disease (DOHaD) was established to promote research into the fetal origins of disease and involves scientists from many backgrounds. There is some evidence that pregnant women with allergies have modified immune interactions with their fetus compared to other pregnant women who don't have allergies, and that these allergic moms-to-be are more likely to have infants with food allergies.

Two 2016 studies published in the influential journal *Science Translational Medicine* have suggested that signs of food allergies may be present already at birth in immune cells, such as monocytes, a type of white blood cell. In one of those studies, the umbilical cord blood of Australian infants who later developed food allergies was loaded with overactive versions of monocytes—suggesting that these soon-to-be food-allergic children already had altered immune function by the time they were born. They also had epigenetic changes that were associated with food allergies. It has been insinuated that those overexcited cells may push other immune cells to become allergy-causing cells. And yet, genetics aren't entirely to blame.

A 2013 study in *JAMA Pediatrics* found that foreign-born children who immigrate to the US have a lower risk of developing allergies than their US-born peers. Specifically: 20 percent of foreign-born kids in America developed allergic diseases compared with 34 percent of the American-born children with foreign-born parents. The prevalence of asthma was even lower, with those born outside the US 47 percent less likely to develop the condition than those born in the US. Put simply, the children who were born in their country of origin and immigrated with their parents to the US were almost half as likely to develop allergic diseases than were their American-born counterparts with immigrant parents. The interesting twist, revealed by subsequent studies, is when these foreign-born children grow up and have their own kids born in the US, these second-generation immigrant children have a greater risk of food allergy, not just compared to their parents, but also compared to their US-born peers. I know this personally as my family is a perfect example. I immigrated with my parents at age two and have no allergic conditions. My two kids, however, are highly allergic, both with allergic rhinitis and one with food allergies.

What was the environmental protection they lost in those first years of life? Even after the researchers accounted for factors that could affect rates of allergies, such as race, ethnicity, and/or socioeconomic status, the strong association between being born in the US and the higher risk of allergic diseases remained. My own investigations have confirmed this pattern. Different environments appear to flip the allergy switch (much more on this in Chapter 5).

This is true for adults who unexpectedly develop food allergies. A move to a new state or country with different allergens can be an instigator. Changes in geography usually involve changes in the environment, including native plants and pollutants that can bring on allergies for the first time at any age. What's more, different environmental factors can cross-react with ingredients (mostly proteins) in food; for example, adult-onset allergy to shellfish (shrimp, lobster) can be related to a hidden, previously undiagnosed allergy to dust mites or cockroaches—the two share a relationship due to similar proteins present in the muscles of these leggy creatures.

According to a study in a November 2017 issue of the *Journal of Allergy and Clinical Immunology*, 42 percent of adults with atopic dermatitis (eczema), for example, developed it in adulthood, most commonly on their hands, head, or neck. Additionally, in our study, 50 percent of adults with food allergy reported at least one new food allergy developing as an adult. It helps to understand that immune systems are dynamic—

they change and evolve with us as we encounter new environments and exposures. The immune system you have today is not identical to the one you had a decade ago, nor will it be the same a decade from now. Such dynamism is why some of the theories behind adult-onset allergies revolve around exposure to allergens when the immune system is weakened, such as during an illness, pregnancy, or prolonged period of stress (in general, the immune system weakens with age, which explains why older adults are more vulnerable to such illnesses as shingles and pneumonia). Infectious agents, for instance, viruses, can adversely tweak the immune system, provoking it to respond incorrectly to otherwise safe food proteins. Hormonal changes during puberty, pregnancy, and menopause also can tip the immune system's behavior in favor of reacting to certain foods. In fact, people who go through oral immunotherapy for food allergy sometimes have to factor in their hormonal cycles into their treatment, as fluctuations—especially in women after menopause and in pubescent girls—can respond differently. And then there's the possibility that someone who is not exposed to a high enough level of the allergen to elicit an allergic reaction as a child finally reaches that threshold in adulthood.

Remember: nearly half—a whopping 48 percent—of adults with food allergies developed at least one *in adulthood*; and, as with children, the incidence of food allergies in adults appears to be rising across all ethnic groups. When I published this data in 2019, I noted that the most common food allergy among US adults is shellfish, affecting an estimated 2.9 percent of US adults. This marks an increase from the 2.5 percent prevalence rate published in an influential 2004 study. Similarly, these new data suggest that adult tree nut allergy prevalence has risen to 1.8 percent from a 2008 estimate of 0.5 percent, an increase of 260 percent. That amounts to nearly 4.5 million people. For some, the adult-onset allergy can last a lifetime. Unlike children who can outgrow some of their food allergy, that's less likely to happen to adults. Consequently, learning to live with food allergy and avoid food allergens during daily life becomes paramount.

RAGING HORMONES: CAN I BE ALLERGIC TO MY OWN HORMONES?

Hormones are biological messengers produced in glands, such as the pituitary, adrenal, ovaries, and testes, that travel through the blood to other parts of the body, where they exert their effects. More than fifty different hormones and related molecules regulate nearly every bodily process and are critical to the function of almost every tissue, organ, and system. Hormones regulate your metabolism, growth and development between birth and maturity, tissue function, fluid balance, blood pressure, fertility, moods, response to injury, stress, environmental factors, and much more.

The ones you probably know easily by name are those tied to sex and reproduction: progesterone, testosterone, and estrogen. In the past decade, a rare condition called progestogen hypersensitivity (a.k.a. autoimmune progesterone dermatitis) has entered the medical lexicon. It affects women of childbearing years who experience a recurrence of itchy, blisterlike skin rashes in a cyclical manner corresponding to their menstrual cycle. They may also have abdominal pain, flushing, fatigue, and shortness of breath. Although exceedingly rare, anaphylaxis has also been reported with this condition, which is thought to be an autoimmune-driven allergic reaction to one's own progesterone during the phase of the cycle when this hormone is elevated. Doctors attuned to this new diagnosis can treat with certain medications to dampen ovarian function (and the release of hormones) to prevent and better manage those reactions. I bring up this uncommon masquerader because not only is it unrelated to food, but it also speaks to the intricacy of the human body. And in the next chapter, we'll explore more about the hidden connections between allergic diseases and autoimmunity. It's now a fascinating, growing field of study.

Although allergic diseases have a genetic component and are more prevalent in individuals with a family history of the conditions, the dramatic rise in documented allergic diseases cannot be explained by changes in relatively static genes alone. As the surge in allergic disease has occurred more rapidly than alterations to the actual genome can occur (it takes many multiple generations—sometimes millions of years—for such changes to happen), and because allergic disease appears significantly more prevalent in Westernized countries, it has been hypothesized that certain relatively recent modifications to our dietary habits, lifestyle, and surrounding environment are responsible for the increased prevalence of allergic disease across the spectrum at every age.

The current, most talked-about factors linked with the allergy epidemic include three powerful culprits: changes in early-life microbial exposures; dietary factors (e.g., late introduction to certain foods in infancy, shifts in modern farming practices and food manufacturing, an increased pro-inflammatory modern diet); and exposure to pollutants associated with urbanization (i.e., cars and traffic that create a lot of pro-inflammatory particulates in the air). These shifts in modern life foment a perfect storm for people living in the twenty-first century. And we'll focus on the first two, since they dominate in research circles.

YOUR MICROBIAL FRIENDS HELP SHAPE YOUR IMMUNITY

Sanitation and cleanliness have substantially improved our health over the past century, and regular hand washing and daily bathing are a big part of that (especially during acute periods, such as what we've experienced with the coronavirus pandemic). But aside from the exceptions brought on by Covid-19, we could be paying a price for an excessive overall clean-up in the past century. Very few of us are exposed to potential adversaries to the immune system early on in life (and throughout) that challenge our immune system and essentially fortify it against allergies. Not many of us live on farms, are routinely exposed to animals and pets as was more common in earlier generations, or even play outdoors much anymore. Our contemporary lifestyle keeps many of us indoors, "germ-free," and missing out on opportunities to commune with nature in healthy ways that help to "educate" and support our immune system that can desensitize us to common environmental allergens. And when we do venture outside our sealed buildings, it's often within artificial contexts with minimal biodiversity, such as concrete playgrounds and large fields planted with commercial, nonnative grass or artificial turf.

In 1989, the British epidemiologist David Strachan was the first to suggest the "Hygiene Hypothesis" that exposure to infections during childhood would provide a good defense against allergies in later life. He proposed that a lower incidence of infection in early childhood could be an explanation for the twentieth-century uptick in allergic diseases. In the *British Medical Journal*, Strachan published his findings that children in larger households had fewer instances of hay fever because they are exposed to germs by older siblings. This led to further research suggesting that a lack of early childhood exposure to less than pristine conditions can increase the individual's susceptibility to disease. Although a simple idea in itself, it raised the theory that rising incidences of chronic allergic disease may be an inevitable price to be paid for freedom from the burden of killer infectious diseases.

The idea is similar to what happens when a person builds muscle mass and strength through weight training. To be able to lift heavy objects, you have to work your muscles by gradually increasing the weight of the objects you lift. Without proper training, you won't be able to lift a heavy object on demand. The same is thought to be true for the immune system. To fight off infection (a "weight" of sorts), the immune system must train by fighting off contaminants found in everyday life. Systems that aren't exposed to contaminants have trouble with the heavy lifting of fighting off infections.

This conversation wouldn't be complete without a deeper discussion about the relationship between our immune system and our microbiome—the collection of all the microbes living on and inside the body, many of which support our health and share a powerful, mutually beneficial relationship with our body. The microbiome is the link—the biological hinge, if you will—that connects your interactions with your environment (and potential allergens) and immune system. You've probably heard about the human microbiome by now, as much has been written about it, but trying to fully understand it might still give you pause.

The term *microbiome* comes from the combination of *micro*, for "supersmall" or "microscopic," and *biome*, which refers to a naturally occurring community of life-forms occupying a large habitat, in this case the human body. When I began to study immunology and microbiology as a medical student, nobody could tell you what a microbiome was; today, decoding our microbiome—from the communities deep inside our guts to the colonies that cover our skin—is one of the most promising fields of scientific study. We are at the very beginning of an exciting journey to understanding—and leveraging the power of—the human microbiome.

The ecosystem that comprises a human biome includes a diverse collection of microorganisms, mainly bacteria, fungi, yeasts, parasites, and viruses. Their collective genetic material far outnumbers our own DNA. The current thinking is that, whereas some microbes might reach us while we're still in our mothers' womb, the majority of the initial colonization happens when we descend through the birth canal and are exposed to organisms living there. These microbes shower over us, causing our microbiome to bloom at birth. The process continues as we begin life in the outside world. This may, by the way, help explain the difference between the lifetime health of babies born vaginally and the health of those born via a relatively sterile C-section. The science now shows that C-section babies may not develop the right microbiome and, as a result, can have a higher risk for certain conditions later in life—mostly inflammatory, metabolic, and immune problems (yes, asthma and food allergies included). The jury is still out, however, about whether missing out on the microbial baptism at birth from a C-section can be overcome with other strategies to protect the baby and provide support to the healthy development of the microbiome. Many factors contribute to a baby's microbiome and lifetime risk for certain diseases, method of birth being just one. Other factors include the mother's health and age, breast-feeding status, early life exposures, and dietary habits.

"WAS IT MY FAULT?"

When a woman gives birth to a child that develops serious food allergies, and for sake of this conversation, let's throw eczema and asthma into the mix as well, it's common for a mother to start wondering if she's to blame. I have heard this so frequently (and honestly have wondered about it myself with my children). Was it the diet she followed during pregnancy? Something she was exposed to? Her unplanned cesarean section? Absolutely not!

Let's get one thing straight: The best studies and the majority of publications to date support the conclusion that avoiding certain foods during pregnancy, breastfeeding, or both are not effective in preventing allergic disease. A 2012 systematic review including five randomized trials and over nine hundred patients also reached this conclusion. But some moms-to-be are not getting the message. In a 2018 analysis of data from 4,900 pregnant women, about 3 percent of these expectant mothers reported cutting back on nuts, eggs, and dairy in the hope of preventing food allergies in their newborn.

The C-section factor, however, does give us reason to pause and debate further. In 2016, a group of Greek researchers found that cesarean section predicted food allergy among 459 children examined at eight intervals during their first three years of life. Babies delivered this way and with at least one food-allergic parent were more likely to develop their own allergy than were those delivered vaginally and whose parents were not allergic (which factor mattered, the delivery or the inherited allergy, is unclear). Food allergy was also more common during the first two years of life among 2,500 German infants born via C-section. And a Swedish study of more than one million births between 2001 and 2012 found a 21 percent higher risk of food allergy among C-section babies compared to those born by vaginal delivery.

The reason may not be due solely to the C-section, however. It likely lies in a confluence of factors, starting with the effects a natural vaginal birth has on a baby's developing microbiome. A baby moving through the birth canal is "baptized" by microbes that then go on to help train the immune system. Babies born via a sterile C-section miss out on the party. But this data should not be translated to mean expectant mothers must always avoid C-sections or that C-section dooms a baby to develop health challenges as a result. A lot of other factors contribute to the development of food allergy (or any health condition) that come into the picture long after birth, such as antibiotic uses, environmental exposures, early food introduction, and so on. Cesareans are medically necessary under many circumstances and serve an important role in medicine.

Just to reiterate: It's not worth playing the blame game. We all are doing the best with what we know right now. There are so many factors at play. I was interviewed by a national newspaper and asked about the early peanut introduction study as an expert. I was then asked about my daughter and what I had done. The article said something to the effect of "Dr. Gupta is slapping herself on the wrist for not introducing peanut to her daughter earlier." Do not ever feel guilty for undergoing a C-section. Guilt is everywhere. Let it go and keep doing your best!

The bacteria that thrive in our intestines are especially important. They have a commanding say in everything about us, from the efficiency and speed of our metabolism to our risk for all manner of ills, allergic conditions among them. They assist with digestion and the absorption of nutrients; you can't nourish yourself effectively without them. They also make and release important enzymes and other substances that your body requires but cannot make sufficiently on its own. These include vitamins (notably B vitamins) and neurotransmitters, such as dopamine and serotonin. An estimated 90 percent of the feel-good hormone serotonin in your body is not made in your brain. It's produced in your digestive tract, thanks to your gut bugs. Your "intestinal flora," as it's also called, and their effects on your hormonal system help you handle stress and even get a good night's sleep. Okay, so that's the quick 101 on gut bacteria (a whole book can be written—and many have— on this subject alone). Let's get to the connection with food allergies. The relationship between your microbes and immune system reflects your body's center of gravity for the likelihood of your suffering from food allergies.

Microbial Meddling in Immunity

My colleague Christina Ciaccio, MD, Chief of Allergy and Immunology and Associate Professor at the University of Chicago where she's a prominent researcher on the microbiome, is developing treatments that modify the microbiome to help prevent and treat food allergy. She notes that the dramatic multigenerational changes to the microbiome that we've seen has no doubt been caused by our environment. Over the past thirty years or so, we can also see an equally dramatic change to the prevalence of food allergy. Dr. Ciaccio and others believe that the shift in our microbiome has also affected our risk for food allergies due to the relationship our resident microbiota has with our physiology.

You see, of all the actions that these microscopic organisms perform to keep you healthy, perhaps the most vital are the ones that regulate and support your immune system, which is tied directly to your risk for allergic diseases. We live in symbiosis with the bacteria in our guts. They give us something to stay healthy, and we give them something like fibrous fruits and vegetables so they can stay healthy. Perhaps most important when talking about food allergy and related conditions, these microbes also help the immune system accurately distinguish between friend and foe.

Under normal circumstances, they decide what should be safe, such as food. Remember how important Dr. Lack thinks it is for food to first get introduced to the immune system through the mouth and gut? We may not be holding up our end of the bargain, however. Many of our eating and cleaning habits have changed over the past several generations, so understanding the microbiome, and how we have disrupted it, may be critical to how we explain the disturbing increase in allergic and autoimmune diseases in the Western world.

Our diet and cleaning habits are just two of the things that have changed over the past several generations that may have caused our microbiomes to shift away from those bacteria that are so good at controlling our immune system. For example, we ingest antibiotics (both prescribed and those occasionally found in our food and, to a lesser extent, water supply, as a result of industrial agriculture) now more than ever before. We've decreased exposure to pathogens and infections due to sanitation and public health measures (a remarkable achievement with possible side effects nonetheless). We've changed our housing to less densely inhabited and cleaner buildings. We've largely moved away from farms and into cities and suburbs. And, of course, we have a higher incidence of births via C-sections followed by formula feeding. We do not want to minimize the profound effect that the shift in our diet has had either. The standard American diet is composed of nutrient poor, low fiber, highly processed foods high in sugar and the wrong fats. According to Dr. Ciaccio, "Small dietary changes cause an almost immediate change in our microbiomes." And she adds: "We do not expect our environment to suddenly shift back to what it was for our great-grandparents. We don't want many of the changes to shift back. We are looking for ways to work around this."

Many of the changes that have been made are not inherently bad— C-sections, infant formula, and sanitization save lives in many circumstances. Even the shifts in our food production have created better, more reliable access to food. But these shifts do have profound effects on our microbiome that we cannot ignore. Dr. Ciaccio hopes to find strategies that can reintroduce key fibers, microbes, and molecules into the gut that support the natural strength and function of one's microbiome, which is like a satellite organ of the immune system.

Because gut bacteria can control certain immune cells and help manage the body's inflammatory pathways, the gut (including its inhabitants) is said to be your immune system's largest "organ." You may even know already that the skin is the largest physical organ. Biologically speaking, the gut and the skin are one and the same, as they present barriers between our insides and outsides that are colonized with microbes that can help and hinder their performance (in fact, the skin and intestinal lining share similar origins in utero during embryonic development). The immune system is dynamic and ever-changing alongside the microbiome throughout our lifetime.

Indeed, we humans are essentially large, complex ecosystems, where the microbes that live on and within us constitute an organ at least as essential to health as our liver or kidneys. It helps to think of the immune system as a learning device, and at birth it resembles a computer with hardware and software but scant data. Additional data must be supplied during the first years of life, through contact with microorganisms from other humans and the natural environment. If these inputs are inadequate or inappropriate, the regulatory mechanisms of the immune system can fail. As a result, the system attacks not only harmful organisms that cause infections but also innocuous targets, such as pollen, house dust, and food proteins, resulting in allergic diseases.

Many researchers have now confirmed that exposure to a little "dirt"—through siblings and other housemates, growing up on a farm or living in a developing country—can be beneficial and even ward off disease, thanks to the effects on the microbiome. In 2014, a team led by Dr. Cathryn Nagler, Bunning family professor at the University of Chicago, published a landmark study showing that Clostridia perfringens, a common class of gut bacteria, protects against certain food allergies. When the researchers fed peanut allergens to germ-free mice (born and raised in sterile conditions) and to mice treated with antibiotics as newborns (reducing their gut bacteria), the animals showed a strong immunological response. This sensitization could be reversed, however, by reintroducing Clostridia perfringens—but not another class of bacteria, Bacteroides—into the mice. Further experiments revealed that Clostridia caused immune cells to produce high levels of interleukin-22 (IL-22), a signaling molecule known to decrease the permeability of the intestinal lining. "In simple terms," Nagler says, "what we found is that these bacteria prevent food allergens from gaining access to the blood in an intact form that elicits an allergic reaction."

In another study the following year not involving Nagler, and which capped decades of observations, researchers quantified the reduction in risk of asthma for children growing up with dogs. The investigators combed through the records of more than one million children born in Sweden between 2001 and 2010. Of the 275,000 or so school-age children in the cohort, the researchers found that the children of dog-owning families had a 13 percent lower chance of developing asthma than did their peers who grew up without a dog.

The idea that pets can enhance the microbiome makes even more sense when viewed in light of the Old Friends, or Microbiome, Hypothesis, a refinement of the Hygiene Hypothesis. In this view, humans' coevolution with livestock and animals has made us dependent on their microbes for our health and even survival. Losing contact with these "old friends" might tip the delicate evolutionary balance.

In dermatology, doctors talk a lot about what's called the atopic march, sometimes referred to as the allergic march, and which could be related to the Hygiene Hypothesis. We often see a natural progression—a "march"—of diagnoses in early life: first atopic dermatitis (eczema) in the first six months of life, then asthmalike symptoms beginning between the ages of two and four, and finally allergic rhinitis (hay fever) in school-age children. Food allergies can also emerge between ages one and two that are directly related to the march. A steep rise in the number of people, usually children, who suffer from one or more of these conditions has resulted in investigations that led scientists like me to determine that excessive cleanliness in a child's environment may be partly to blame. We also postulate, as I've already highlighted, that controlling or preventing eczema early on, which is often the first sign of a food allergy problem down the road, may be a preventive strategy.

All that aside, being "too clean" and infection-free does not tell the whole story. It is certainly important that we are colonized with some bacteria and not infected by others. In fact, there is a campaign within the medical community to phase out the term "Hygiene Hypothesis" because it can be misleading and overly simplify what is undoubtedly a complex interplay of factors that are fueling the rise in food allergies.

Connecting More Dots

In 2016, my team published a paper that somewhat altered the prevailing wisdom and that has been substantiated by other scientists in the field. Missing out on early exposure to a panoply of substances that challenge the immune system—and essentially setting it up for life—is not the only mechanism behind the rise in food allergies. As Gideon Lack documented, there is also something to be said for exposure to a food allergen *through broken skin*, which then prompts the development of food allergy. This theory gained further support from another study that found increased prevalence of food allergy if a child had a skin infection or eczema in the first year of life (more evidence that alleviating eczema could have long-term protective effects in food allergy).

Our study recruited 1,359 participants, from birth to twenty-one years old, with and without food allergies. What made this family-based study particularly unique is that it included siblings who may or may not have had allergies. The similar genetic makeup of the kids and controls helped us assess the impact of different exposures on food allergy and asthma. We investigated key hygiene factors in association with food allergy and asthma, including antibiotic use, infection history, number of siblings, pet exposure, and maternal/child health factors, such as maternal age at birth, cesarean section, breastfeeding, and out-of-home childcare. And when it comes to early childhood settings, kids in daycare environments are exposed to more germs that also confer immune-boosting benefits and food allergy protection in the long run.

The number of siblings and children in a childcare center were the only hygiene factors that were associated with decreased food allergy (more kids, less allergies). This was an important finding. It strengthened the idea that the exposure to multiple kids and consequently potential bacteria, viruses, and microbiome play a critical role in the early potential protection against the development of food allergies.

It is so important to note that the development of food allergies do not revolve around a single smoking gun. Just as there are multiple ways an individual can develop cancer that entail both underlying genetics and overlying environmental ingredients, there are diverse mechanisms behind the development of food allergies, some of which we just don't know about yet. A constellation of events likely happens in people susceptible to food allergies—one that has both genetic and environmental forces acting in sync.

Some of my other research has revealed interesting nuances to the allergy story. Children who live in a community with a lot of violent and drug-related crime experience more asthma, with rates as high as 44 percent in Chicago's South and West Sides. (Remember: Generally speaking, children diagnosed with asthma also commonly have food allergies.) While we don't know all the mechanisms for why this is so, my educated guess is we'll find that living under such stressful conditions has downstream effects on the immune system through shared inflammatory pathways (see next chapter). Socioeconomic factors could also be contributing to risk, as people with lower economic means may live in places where they could be exposed to more environmental toxins, from mold in old buildings to air pollution near heavily trafficked city centers and highways.

The work of my colleague Dr. Katie Allen, formerly of the Murdoch Research Institute in Australia, and now a member of the Australian parliament, has brought to light another clue to consider: vitamin D.

Or, more precisely, lack of this important vitamin.* Vitamin D, some-times called the "sunshine vitamin," is a nutrient—a hormone—essential for good health. It plays a major role in the maintenance of healthy bones by helping the body absorb calcium, and also has a critical role in immune system function. Sufficient levels help protect against all manner of diseases, from type 1 diabetes and hypertension to cancer, autoimmune ailments, and allergic diseases. Most recently, vitamin D deficiency has been linked to severe risk of Covid-19 infection and may increase the mortality risk 3.7-fold in hospitalized patients. Even the health and function of your heart, lungs, and brain rely on this nutrient. It's no wonder that evolution allowed us to make this vitamin easily through simple sunlight exposure. The rise in food allergy runs parallel with increased prevalence of vitamin D deficiency in pregnancy (and in the community generally), but we don't know whether this is a cause or if other factors occurring during the child's first year of life are to blame.

The fact, however, that vitamin D factors mightily into the strength and function of the immune system speaks volumes. It also communicates with the microbiome in ways that fortify the developing and constantly evolving immune system. If enough vitamin D is not available, perhaps irregularities in the system can occur. I find it telling that Dr. Allen's studies have found that children deficient in vitamin D may be more likely to have a food allergy. They are also more likely to have multiple food allergies. My guess is we will continue to document connections between vitamin D status and risk for allergic diseases (among other ailments) across all ages, adults included. It's estimated that 50 percent of the population in Western countries may lack sufficient levels of vitamin D, with 10 percent of people clinically deficient in this important vitamin. Even Dr. Anthony Fauci, director of the NIAID, recommends vitamin D to support a decrease in Covid-19 severity and complications.

---

*Dr. Allen has cleverly organized the main categories of current hypotheses into the 5 Ds: diet, dogs, vitamin D, dry skin, and dirt. We'll be returning to these chief influencers in Part 2.

These estimations, however, come with a caveat: This is a dynamic area of study that will gain more clarity and data in the future. There's no universal consensus, for example, regarding the definition of "insufficiency" and even testing for vitamin D levels (and what those numbers truly mean) has been a source of debate. Although the research comparing vitamin D deficiencies to food allergies is not conclusive and we don't know whether vitamin D can reverse food allergies, what we do know is vitamin D may protect against allergic diseases and is necessary for overall health and well-being.

We get most of our vitamin D from the exposure to UV sunlight, which triggers a cascade of events in the skin to manufacture this hormone. Fully 80 to 90 percent of your vitamin D levels come from sun exposure. Inadequate exposure to sunlight, rather than diet, is the most common cause of low vitamin D levels, as vitamin D is present in only very low amounts in most foods. Some studies have shown that areas farther away from the equator (and thus with lower ambient ultraviolet radiation) have higher rates of childhood food allergy–related hospital admissions, epinephrine autoinjector prescriptions, and peanut allergy (up to six times the risk) than areas closer to the equator. Season of birth (being born in autumn or winter when there is less UV exposure) has also been associated with higher risk of anaphylaxis and food allergy.

Don't dismay though, if you are like me and live in a colder environment (Chicago). In a geographic food allergy paper we published, we did not see this variation in the US—and in fact living at lower latitudes was not associated with reduced risk of food allergy. The main association we found in our study was that urban areas had higher rates of food allergy compared to rural areas, which does still put me in a higher risk area after all.

However, in Australia, a growing number of studies have identified compelling links between vitamin D and food allergy risk. One particularly striking longitudinal study of Australian children published in 2012 found a dose-response relationship between lower latitude and greater food allergy risk, extending previous work finding similar associations between lower latitude and higher rates of epineph-rine autoinjector prescriptions—an indicator of physician-diagnosed food allergy.

A link between late introduction of egg, one of the few common dietary sources of vitamin D in the infant diet, and food allergy has been documented in a large Australian study. Infants who were first fed egg earlier (between four and six months) had significantly less food allergy than infants first fed egg later (after six months of age).

The vitamin D component to the food allergy mystery is vigorously debated today. More recent research has challenged the vitamin D theory, again largely because we lack a standard definition for vitamin D defi-ciency and we don't know what "optimal" level may be needed to impact immune function. It's a provocative theory, nonetheless, and one I want to bring up. It could very well be that the association points to other, more significant factors that help explain the food allergy epidemic. And with that in mind, let's turn to matters of diet. And this is where food intolerances come into the picture in addition to food allergies.

DIETARY DEFECTS AND EVOLUTIONARY MISMATCH

You are what you eat. This is especially true when it comes to the compo-sition of your microbiome. If there's one thing we scientists have learned in just the last decade or so, it's that changes in diet result in adjust-ments to our microbiota. As our ancestors' diet evolved over time, their gut inhabitants did, too, from microbes that could easily break down the fibrous foods plentiful in the early human diet to other microbes better-equipped to process the animal proteins, sugars, and starches prevalent after the advent of agriculture and animal husbandry about ten thousand years ago. But as we all know, Westerners have taken the consumption of animal protein, sugars (especially overly refined), and starches to the extreme. We love our burgers, cereals, bagels, pizzas, and processed foods. And the result is a diet high in empty calories and deficient in such nutrients as fiber, essential fatty acids, and other micronutrients that help nourish a healthy microbiome and, in turn, a strong immune system. As the saying goes, we are overfed and undernourished. New research suggests that people living in rural Africa, whose eating patterns more closely resemble our ancestors', have a healthier mix of microbes in their gut than do their Western counterparts, which may protect them from many of the ills that are common in modern developed countries, from food allergies and intolerances to intestinal diseases, autoimmune disorders, and even neurodegenerative ailments, such as Alzheimer's disease.

The idea that we eat counter to what our DNA expects is sometimes referred to as the evolutionary mismatch theory. Although this one is hard to prove due to a lack of long-term data to date and the kind of double-blind, placebo-controlled studies that are common in other areas of medicine, it's a compelling concept nonetheless that dovetails with the Microbiome Hypothesis and which future research will help us better understand. It's mentioned specifically with regard to food allergies, so let's cover that first within the context of the immune system's development.

From a purely evolutionary perspective, allergic reactions are not necessarily immune system mistakes—they are an adaptive response to potentially damaging environmental exposures. The allergic response evolved to help us deal with potential insults to the body, from substances in food and chemicals to other living things, such as intestinal parasites. But by many measures, some of our immune systems are "mistaken"—they are reacting to foods that they really shouldn't, given our evolutionary history and normal physiology. These allergic reactions are unnecessarily exaggerated and maladaptive. The immune system's ability to be properly *tolerant* of foods has been subjected to natural selection for millions of years. It should not be prone to frequent overreaction. And therein lies the key word: *tolerance*. And being "tolerant" to all kinds of foods has everything to do with the microbiome and its training grounds during its development and ongoing transformation. Let me explain.

From the sterile environment of the womb, the newborn infant is exposed to a vast array of new foreign substances (antigenic proteins) in relatively high "doses." Most of this antigenic load is actually derived from those colonizing commensal bacteria and food components that come through the mother in the form of breastmilk (or formula) and surrounding environmental inputs. To prevent inflammatory responses to these largely harmless antigens, the gut's surrounding immune system, what's called the gastrointestinal-associated lymphoid tissue (GALT) has evolved complex mechanisms to promote tolerance as a default response. In other words, its built-in technology knows how to handle these exposures without triggering an adverse immune response. At least 80 percent of our body's total immune system is made up of GALT. Our immune system is headquartered in the gut because the intestinal wall is a biological gateway of sorts to the outside world, so aside from skin, it's where we have the greatest chance of encountering foreign material and organisms. The GALT is in constant communication with every other immune-system cell throughout the body, notifying them if cells in the gut encounter a potentially harmful substance.

Children alive in the Paleolithic era who reached the age of one year or perhaps a little older would have been exposed to most or perhaps even all of the different types of food antigens they would ever be exposed to in their lifetime. This stands in sharp contrast to the children of today who live in developed countries. These kids are at risk of an unprecedented degree of "mismatch" between early and late food antigen exposures. In other words, what they are exposed to in utero and soon after birth is removed from what they encounter later on in life as they develop and grow into adults. Such a disconnect creates a mismatch, and they lose an opportunity to build up their tolerance. Food allergies in the immune system's reflexive response to this discord are the potential consequence.

New parents in the Western world used to be given a list of foods to avoid for their baby due to the fear that their child would have a reaction and become allergic to these foods. This had the unfortunate effects of limiting a fetus and baby's exposure to potential allergens that could prime the immune system and prevent the development of the allergy. As the guidelines have not been fully adapted, some families still adhere to those rules. And, after birth, by shielding their babies from exposure to a diverse array of foods once they venture beyond breast milk, they could inadvertently be setting them up to suffer the consequences as they grow up in the form of severe food allergies.

Now, the thinking has totally reversed, and multiple studies have confirmed that indeed, early and frequent exposure to a diverse array of foods is beneficial to living an allergy-free life. The data for peanut is clear and our Center for Food Allergy & Asthma Research (CFAAR) is in the process of determining whether the same applies for other common food allergens, such as milk, egg, tree nuts, soy, and sesame. We are working with researchers around the world on this and will have answers soon.

Drugs as Biome Influencers

Some of our modern conveniences, namely pharmaceuticals, can have an impact on our microbiome too. If medicines such as antibiotics or acid-reducing stomach medication are overused, especially early in life, those changes to the gastrointestinal tract's microbiome can create more immune-based confusion and health-related problems—including not only food allergies but also metabolic challenges and even autoimmune disorders.

The influence of medications cannot be underestimated, especially among adults who have a daily regimes to manage conditions over the long term. Granted, these medications are often necessary and beneficial for the purposes they serve, but we cannot neglect the side effects they may have on the microbiome that, in turn, raise risk for allergic diseases. In 2019, a group of researchers from the Netherlands warned that as many as half of all commonly used drugs profoundly affect the gut microbiome, suggesting that such changes could increase the risk of serious conditions. In particular, they found that eighteen common drug categories were associated with changes in the composition or function of the gut microbiome.

The categories with the biggest impact? Some of the most popular, blockbuster medicines today: proton pump inhibitors (e.g., stomach acid reducers, such as Prilosec and Prevacid), metformin (the prevailing diabetes drug used to help control blood sugar), antibiotics, laxatives, antidepressants, and oral steroids. Many people take more than one of these medications on a regular basis. Although much of the concerns about these drugs' insults to the health and function of the microbiome has largely centered on downstream effects on metabolism and risk for, say, diabetes or an intestinal disorder, now that we know how close the relationship is between the microbiome and immune system, allergic diseases must also be brought into this investigative work and dialogue. A question we need to answer: How much does a person's regular use of certain medications influence risk for developing an allergic disease or intolerance, perhaps suddenly? Some studies are starting to reveal that antacids and antibiotics are among the most powerful grenades in increasing risk for allergic diseases, especially when they are overly used. And, as you probably know, these are popular drugs dispensed daily to both children and adults. In Part 2, I'll caution against reflexively asking for these prescriptions when they are truly unnecessary.

Although the microbiome has a powerful relationship with the immune system, which is partly why any conversation about food allergies must eventually mention the microbiome, my guess is the dialogue will soon widen to include intolerances. As you know, these reactions are not immune-based but we are increasingly learning more about how the microbiome lords over much of our physiology, including its digestive powers, metabolism, hormonal system, and inflammatory pathways. It's in constant conversation with the brain through the vagus nerve— what's called the gut-brain axis. Any food, for example, that causes intestinal distress or headaches no doubt involves biochemical exchanges between these microbial cells and our own. Gut bacteria make chemicals that communicate with the brain through nerves and hormones; the communication is a unique and complex network. So, not only is the gut's community key to immunity, but it's also a linchpin to our entire nervous system.

It's logical to see how a shift in the health and composition of our microbiome in the modern era has contributed to more people enduring challenging relationships with food. The microbiome's connection to the immune system and digestive system means it serves double duty: it mediates how our immune and digestive systems function and react—or not—to certain foods. Microbiome projects are well under way around the world, as this area of medicine is still in its infancy. Although there is still much to learn, it is quite clear that the gut microbiome plays an important role in countless physical and psychological processes. My hope is that in the future we will learn how to tweak the microbiome to not only prevent and treat allergies but eradicate intolerances too.

Fearless Facts

→ Early dietary exposure in life to a diverse array of foods when babies begin to eat solid foods (i.e., between four and six months of age) helps prevent the development of food allergy; the longer you wait to introduce certain allergenic foods like peanuts, the greater the potential risk for developing allergies to those foods.

→ Compromised skin in a baby, due to such conditions as severe eczema, is a significant risk factor to developing food allergy. Infants with severe eczema need to be evaluated early by an allergist and, if recommended, start eating peanut-containing products to prevent peanut allergy.

→ Although certain genes have been linked with higher risk for food allergies, immigration patterns and changes in allergy prevalence also show the power of different environmental factors that can flip the allergy switch.

→ The immune system is dynamic, so forces that change its behavior—from infections to hormonal cycles across the life span—can lead to shifts in risk for allergies and related food conditions.

→ Our microbiome, the trillions of microorganisms (also called microbiota or microbes) that include bacteria, fungi, protozoa, and viruses and that live on and inside the human body, profoundly influence the strength and function of our immune system. It is the biological link that connects your interactions with your environment (and potential allergens) and immune system.

→ Overly sanitized, extremely clean environments can fail to provide the necessary diverse exposures to germs required to "educate" the immune system during development so it can learn to distinguish between friend and foe. This may help explain the allergic march seen among children as they are first diagnosed with atopic dermatitis (eczema) in the first six months of life, then food allergies, allergic rhinitis, and asthma. These conditions are related, but not all children have every one of them.

→ Other environmental factors that may impact risk for allergic diseases include vitamin D insufficiency, diet, and medications, such as antibiotics and antacids.

→ Because the microbiome commands much of our physiology, including its digestive powers, metabolism, hormonal system, and inflammatory pathways, it's increasingly being scrutinized and studied for contributing to food sensitivities/intolerances aside from reactions that involve the immune system.

four

INFLAMMATION, ALLERGIES, AUTOIMMUNE DISEASES, AND OTHER AILMENTS

The Hidden Connections of Immune Dysfunction

WITHIN A FEW MONTHS OF TURNING FIFTY IN 2016, JANE HOGAN WENT from being a fit, active, healthy, and happy woman to one who could barely function. This happened after a particularly stressful year that began with the sudden death of her mother from a stroke. Jane started to have joint pain and inflammation migrating throughout her body—from jaw to feet; hands, shoulders, and elbows to toes. She felt as if someone held a voodoo doll of her likeness and was moving those needles around at whim. Nothing about her personal or family history glaringly stood out as a potential culprit, but a few years prior, she'd developed digestive issues with ice cream and a sensitivity to chlorine that made her stop swimming. And she'd chalked up her lifetime bout with excessive gas to a family trait.

The generalized pain that became her proverbial last straw in 2016, however, progressed rapidly over weeks to the point where she had no energy, shuffled when she walked, slept poorly, and found basic self-care difficult from the aches in her hands and grip. The burden of these new struggles took a psychological toll, too, and she hoped to gain control of what was going on before serious depression set in. Her doctor referred her to a rheumatologist and suggested that she try changing her diet while she waited for the appointment, under the thinking that foods could trigger joint pain. At first, Jane thought this was a crazy idea but she was desperate, and the engineer in her went into problem-solving and project manager mode. Within about five days of tweaking her diet, the pain and inflammation subsided by an impressive 50 percent, motivating Jane to learn more about using food as medicine.

Jane was eventually diagnosed with rheumatoid arthritis, an auto-immune disease. Immersing herself in research on autoimmunity, she learned how food and lifestyle can have a huge impact on health and well-being. Granted, Jane was never diagnosed with food allergy or even intolerance (though she suspects she does react to chemicals in processed food), but her experience highlights the profound impact that food can have on the body and its inflammatory pathways and, in turn, immune system. Her dietary regimen today means following a low-FODMAP protocol and limiting most grains, dairy, processed foods, convention-ally raised meats, finfish and shellfish, eggs, sugar, nightshade vegetables (except potato), and legumes. Fruit is limited to mostly berries. She has very little pain and inflammation now. Her experience has been so trans-formative that she's left civil engineering to spread the message from her home in Canada as "the wellness engineer" about the power of food.

Lauren A. is another perfect example of someone who learned the power of food through her own issues with autoimmunity and a mul-titude of food intolerances. A woman in her forties with two children, Lauren has had health issues since kindergarten and does not remember ever "feeling well." She weathered the health storms as a child but by the time she joined UCLA's women's volleyball team in the mid-1990s and struggled to overcome serious pain and fatigue, the diagnoses came in: fibromyalgia and arthritis of the spine (ankylosing spondylitis). These were not easy to identify, and for a brief period Lauren faced skepticism that her symptoms were "all in her head." Unfortunately, such an initial response can be common when there are so many symptoms, some of which can seem vague or unrelated to others, and a lack of iron-clad diagnostic tools. Luckily, Lauren found the right doctor to make the proper diagnoses and her path forward lit up. Since then, she's also been diagnosed with an egg allergy, irritable bowel syndrome (IBS), seasonal allergies, and exercise-induced asthma. She has endured years of chronic fatigue, nausea, headaches, and body pains, but has successfully gotten her pain and fatigue under control. In addition to doctor-prescribed medications to manage her symptoms, Lauren has learned to thrive again with lifestyle changes that help mitigate triggers to reactions and keep inflammation in check. Dietary edits are chief among her strategies—no egg, dairy, corn, or wheat. She tries to maintain a mostly home-cooked diet free of problematic foods that can stoke conditions rooted in inflammation and that trouble her digestive health and metabolism. Regular exercise, yoga, and meditation help too—especially with stress that fans those flames.

Food is often a grand intersection of sorts: it can hurt and it can heal. When we choose what to eat, we choose what information to give our body—information for our cells and tissues all the way down to their molecular structure. Sometimes it helps to move away from the notion that food is just calories for energy ("fuel"), or that food is simply micro-nutrients and macronutrients ("building blocks"). Much to the contrary, food is a tool for *epigenetic* expression, or how your diet and genome interact. This is why underlying genetics can factor into risk for certain conditions, allergic diseases and intolerances included. Your genetics likely participate in every potential diagnosis across the food reaction spectrum.

You probably have not thought about food in this manner before. But the foods you consume send signals from your environment to your DNA. Those signals have the power to change how your genes behave, how your DNA is turned into messages and protein products for your body, and how your resulting biology and physiology operate. And because food is the one piece of information we all have to give our bodies every day, we have to be sure we send the right information that works with our body and supports healthy pathways—not harmful or self-destructive ones.

Jane's and Lauren's individual experiences each entailed different sets of symptoms that could have been interpreted squarely as a food-related condition. But their individual autoimmune conditions—masqueraders, really—were entirely different diagnoses. Yet food became one of their tools they used to nurse themselves back to better health, and to address not only food-related conditions but also their autoimmune challenges. This goes to show how complicated the picture can be, and that there are underlying themes here that do share connections. To be clear: I am not implying that their autoimmune ailments were caused by their diet, or that any diet can render them relieved of their conditions, let alone cured. But these stories do provide interesting insights and anecdotal launchpads for further scientific inquiry.

When people find that avoiding certain foods improves their symptoms despite lack of clear evidence and being able to explain the underlying mechanisms, it is recommended that they consult a physician and registered dietitian to ensure that the remainder of their diet is nutritionally sound. Food reactions combined with any other health conditions, including autoimmune challenges, could reflect hidden connections we have yet to scientifically identify, map out, and understand. After all, food is something we put in our body every day and that has an effect on our biology and the function of all its moving parts. A typical Western diet is increasingly under study for its relationship with a whole host of diseases with shared underlying mechanisms that involve metabolism, immune function, and inflammation. The role of the microbiome increasingly gains real estate in the conversation as well, for we know that the composition and health of the gut's microbiota factor into metabolic and immune function health. Although adverse food reactions and autoimmunity are two separate conversations, they, too, share certain relationships with the body's same metabolism, immune function, and inflammation pathways and in some cases may both be driven by foods.

It's no surprise that when something goes wrong with our health, diet is often among the first things we scrutinize and think about changing. Even in the total absence of a bona fide food allergy or intolerance, food is often a common denominator in the path to wellness. How so? That's what this chapter is all about. I've already given you a primer on the vital collaboration our bodies have with our microbiome and, in turn, immune system. But let's take a closer look, starting with more about our microbial comrades.

IT TAKES GUTS

In the last chapter, I mentioned how the gut-brain axis is a two-way highway. You probably don't think of your gut and brain as being strongly connected as a unit much in the way you see your arms and legs linked up to your brain (and the communication that allows your brain to tell your appendages to move here and there). But you've no doubt experienced this hidden connection through nerve-racking experiences that leave you, for example, feeling sick to your stomach ("butterflies in your stomach") or, worse, running to the bathroom.

The vagus nerve, also known as cranial nerve X and historically cited as the pneumogastric nerve, is the longest of the twelve cranial nerves and is the primary channel of information between the hundreds of millions of nerve cells in your central nervous system and your intestinal nervous system. The name *vagus* is derived from the Latin word for wandering—*vagary*—because this nerve has the longest course of all cranial nerves. (As an aside, there's also an axis to your skin to complete the loop, what's called the gut-brain-skin axis. Hence, when you experience strong emotions, such as fear or embarrassment, your skin may turn "white as a ghost" or flush red.)

Indeed, your nervous system is composed of more than your physical brain and spinal cord. In addition to the central nervous system, you have an intestinal or *enteric* nervous system that is intrinsic to the gastrointestinal tract. Both the central and enteric nervous systems are created from the same tissue during fetal development, and both are connected via that vagus nerve, which extends from the brain stem to the abdomen. It forms part of the involuntary (autonomic) nervous system and directs many bodily processes that don't require conscious thinking, such as maintaining heart rate, breathing, and managing digestion. The sympathetic nervous system is your body's fight-or-flight system—the one that quickens your pulse and blood pressure to shunt blood to your brain and muscles, away from digestion. It keeps you alert and mentally adept. The parasympathetic nervous system, on the other hand, is your rest-and-digest system that allows you to rebuild, repair, and sleep.

In addition to the importance of this vagus nerve to relay messages (and "feelings"), it also helps to know that the health of the gut lining is important—it's what separates your insides from your outsides and all the potential threats that can enter. You see, the gastrointestinal tract is lined with one single layer of surface (epithelial) cells from the esophagus to the anus. In fact, all of the body's mucosal surfaces, including those of the eyes, nose, throat, and gastrointestinal tract, are a large point of entry for various pathogens, so they must be well protected by the body.

The intestinal lining, the largest mucosal surface, has three main functions. First, it serves as the means for the body to obtain nutrients from foods. Second, it blocks the entrance into the bloodstream of potentially harmful particles, chemicals, bacteria, and other organisms and components of organisms that can pose a threat to health. The third function of this cellular barrier is perhaps less well known and deals with its immune function: it contains chemicals called immunoglobulins that bind to bacteria and foreign proteins to prevent them from attaching to the gut's lining. These chemicals are antibodies secreted from immune system cells on the other side of the gut lining, and which are transported into the gut via the intestinal wall. This function ultimately allows such pathogenic organisms and proteins to move on and be excreted.

The body absorbs nutrients from the gut via two pathways. One is the transcellular pathway in which nutrients move or diffuse *through* the epithelial cells; the other is the paracellular pathway in which nutrients pass *between* the epithelial cells. If you're having a hard time visualizing this activity, don't worry about it. The important thing to remember is the following: The dynamic connection between these cells, called a tight junction, reflects an intricate, complicated, and highly regulated system that also involves specialized proteins. When we are talking about permeability issues going on in the gut, a so-called leaky gut, we are referring to problems in the competency of these zipperlike junctions. If they aren't working properly or "unzip," they fail to appropriately patrol what should be allowed to pass. And because they are like gatekeepers—letting potential threats out that will provoke the immune system, guess what: these junctions determine, to a large extent, the level of systemic inflammation. It's well documented now that when an intestinal barrier is compromised somehow and substances from inside the gut can seep to the other side, it can lead to a spectrum of health challenges, including allergic ones.

Here's another key point to remember: intestinal microbes help control your gut's permeability, or how easily substances pass through the intestinal wall that is only one cell thick. Now, having said that, I should also add that even though the cell wall may be one cell thick, the goblet cells produce mucus that attach to the wall and makes the cell wall "thicker." This process of mucus production depends on a back-and-forth interplay with the gut microbiome (the mucus layer has two layers—and the inner mucus layer is renewed every hour). In other words, your gut's microbiota plays a key role in shaping that intestinal barrier structure and factors mightily into its permeability. Microbial imbalances disrupt that wall. And if there are problems with the integrity of those cells that line the gut due to a microbial disturbance, there will be problems with controlling the passage of nutrients from the digestive tube into the body via your circulation.

The term "leaky gut," which scientists prefer to call epithelial damage, used to be viewed as an unproven, dubious theory by conventional researchers and doctors—a scapegoat for a variety of ills. But now an impressive number of well-designed studies have repeatedly shown that when your intestinal barrier is damaged, which again can result in simply having an unhealthy gut flora that cannot protect the integrity of the intestinal lining (called dysbiosis, which literally means "bad mode of life"), you are more susceptible to various conditions—conditions that can emerge as a result of both environmental and genetic forces acting together. Among those often cited in the literature are food intolerances, metabolic dysfunctions (e.g., obesity, diabetes), cardiovascular disorders, dementia, cancer, inflammatory bowel disease, rheumatoid arthritis, asthma, and other autoimmune disease. Even dermatologists are in tune with this gut-brain-skin axis; for example, people who experience sudden adult-onset acne could very well attribute their unwanted skin condition to a broken gut-brain-skin axis. In addition, similar healthy and unhealthy bacteria exist on your skin; this is an area of research by our group and many others. When someone develops what would appear to be wildly different conditions, such as an allergic disease as well as a chronic skin disorder, it wouldn't be absurd to find commonality through these deeply hidden connections. As my colleague, an international leader in dermatology, Dr. Peter Lio states, "We continue to learn that the balance and harmony of the microbiome both on the skin and in the gut play a major role in skin disease. From initially thinking that such changes were simply the result of other factors such as inflammation and skin barrier damage, we now realize that, like dominoes, damaging one part of this intricate and delicate system can cause the other parts to come crashing down. It also helps us understand why simply treating one aspect such as only inflammation often leads to the condition coming back immediately after cessation of the treatment." We work closely with Dr. Lio and Dr. Amy Paller, chair of dermatology at

Northwestern University Feinberg School of Medicine, to better understand the interplay of the skin's own microbiome and the development of allergic conditions.

I should add that the gut's epithelial barrier is not meant to be completely impenetrable, but if it's damaged to the point that inflammation results with changes to the health, strength, and function of the gut microbes, then problems can occur both in the gut and potentially elsewhere in the body. Studies show that increased intestinal permeability, which is not easy to diagnose because there is no gold standard test, may play a role in certain GI conditions, such as celiac, Crohn's disease, and IBS, and scientists are looking into whether it can be associated with autoimmune diseases, such as type 1 diabetes, chronic fatigue syndrome, lupus, and fibromyalgia, among others. Studies are also underway to understand any potential associations between an unhealthy intestinal wall and allergies, asthma, and food intolerances. The relationship between leaky gut (sometimes referred to as leaky gut syndrome) and the risk for developing food allergies and intolerances is now an active area of study. So is the prospect of improving allergic conditions and intolerances through healing intestinal damage. Many doctors do not consider leaky gut to be a legitimate condition, and it has yet to enter the medical lexicon with standards for diagnosing and treating. Same goes for different levels and types of dysbiosis, in which there's an abnormal number of bacteria in the gut or a lack of certain species needed for gut—and, in turn, immune—function to operate ideally. But regardless of the lack of clarity in this realm, it doesn't mean a person's symptoms are any less real. My hunch is with more research to understand the dynamics of the intestinal wall, the gut microbes, immune function, and yes, food reactions, we'll arrive at better language to explain what's going on and how various conditions could be related. For now, theories abound but we need more evidence to draw definitive conclusions.

Suffice it to say, this is not a straightforward science with a one-size-fits-all solution. Because each person has a unique biological "fingerprint," if you will, both food intolerance symptoms and trigger foods are different from one person to another. In other words, in two people who react to MSG, for instance, the popular flavor enhancer in many foods (chiefly Chinese food), the ingredient may cause digestive problems in one person and migraines in another. And in ten migraine patients, there could be ten different sets of trigger foods. The one guilty party all patients will have in common, however, is inflammation.

INFLAMMATION, TAKE TWO

Inflammation is the binding ingredient not only in every chronic disease imaginable, but also in all forms of food allergies and intolerances.

One of the most important discoveries in modern medicine has been the dangers of persistent inflammation. Inflammation is the process underlying every chronic illness and allergic disorder. Inflammation is two-faced: it has a good and a bad side. The good: inflammation helps you recover from illness or injury. As the body's natural healing mechanism, it temporarily amps up the immune system to take care of, say, a skinned knee, a cold virus, or an ingredient in food that it doesn't like. But there's a downside to inflammation. When the process is always "on" and the immune system is permanently keyed up, the biological substances produced during the inflammatory process don't recede, and they begin to harm even healthy cells throughout the body. This type of inflammation is systemic—it's a smoldering disturbance that is usually not confined to one particular area; rather, it affects the entire body. The bloodstream allows it to spread. Fortunately, we have the ability to detect this kind of widespread inflammation through blood tests (e.g., for C-reactive protein [CRP]).

As Chapter 2 detailed, the inflammatory response lies at the heart of an allergic reaction. It's also frequently involved in the response to food intolerances. Painful GI reactions, for instance, to certain ingredients in food may not stimulate the immune system but they can certainly stir up inflammatory responses—otherwise, you wouldn't feel the symptoms, which can be wide and varied. Some of these symptoms, in fact, can mimic other diseases and be a coconspirator for many people with such diagnoses as fibromyalgia, irritable bowel syndrome, GERD (gastroesophageal reflux disease), migraine, attention deficit disorder, arthritis, and even lupus. These conditions share the same underlying problem: rampant inflammation.

Which invites another important question: Do some of our skyrocketing rates of chronic illness rooted in inflammation owe their origins to food-borne responses? Think about that for a moment. I am not implying that any food condition on the spectrum can lead to other serious disorders, but there's something to be said for a body that's constantly under siege by an inflammatory process run amok and how that alone can set one up for other health challenges. Toss in any underlying genetic forces at work that further add weight to the risk for a certain health condition, and you quickly grasp the possibility.

Some of the conditions I just mentioned are autoimmune by nature—they result when a body starts to attack its own normal, healthy cells and tissues by mistake because it's misguided somehow. There's a glitch in the immune system that has it malfunctioning and, ultimately, misbehaving. More than eighty types of autoimmune diseases that affect a wide range of body parts have been documented, from type 1 diabetes, celiac, and inflammatory bowel disease to rheumatoid arthritis, multiple sclerosis, and psoriasis. At the heart of an autoimmune disorder is an abnormal immune response, which is what places these disorders in a parallel universe with food allergies. Indeed, at first glance, allergies and autoimmune disease may seem more different than similar. But both are responses generated by the immune system, and that is where their similarities begin. There are overlaps with cell biology, underlying genetic switches, and resulting inflammatory pathways. In the previous chapter, I briefly described the rare autoimmune disorder that can happen in women who have an allergic reaction to their own ovulation cycle as their body adversely responds to progesterone spikes. Very unusual, but very telling in its lessons about what we have yet to understand about the body's internal cross-talk that reflect profound interrelations.

Research scientists are now trying to figure out whether there are any dots to connect between allergies and autoimmune disease. The biological response may not be identical (in an autoimmune response, tissue destruction occurs; with allergies, the immune system overreacts to harmless allergens), but they are different flavors of reactions that share certain characteristics. What we learn from studying one particular disease can help inform the understanding of another. If we understand, for example, why some people develop fibromyalgia, it will then hopefully be easier to understand why other people may develop lupus. Similarly, if we understand why you are allergic to a food, then maybe that will help us understand why you are allergic to pollen. Integrative knowledge sharing across different areas of medicine and diagnoses is key to learning more about the human body in general and finding new ways to perceive its internal workings.

While we cannot definitively declare that food allergens may also be associated with the development of some autoimmune diseases, the science is just getting underway. In one of the first reports of its kind, scientists at the University of North Carolina School of Medicine showed in 2019 that walnut allergen, in addition to inducing allergic diseases to certain individuals, could also promote autoantibody development in an autoimmune skin disease called pemphigus vulgaris. The chronic skin disorder causes blisters and sores on the skin or mucous membranes (mouth or on the genitals) and is most often seen in people who are middle-aged or older. Such a discovery opens the door now for investigating links between the two major outcomes of a dysfunctional immune system: allergy and autoimmunity. Two entirely different categories of disease sharing a dysregulated immune system.

This is particularly interesting given the 2019 publication of a European study covering more than three million patients, which suggests patients with allergic disease, such as eczema, asthma, and allergic rhinitis, may be at increased risk of developing autoimmune disease later in life. Again, the relationship may not be between allergy and autoimmunity necessarily; rather, a shared issue with an immune system out of healthy order. I can't wait to see how this kind of revolutionary research continues to unfold and clue us all in. At this writing, scientists in the Covid-19 world are trying to decipher why some people who contract the infection go on to suffer from a wide range of symptoms long term. Dubbed "long-haulers," these patients recover from the acute infection but experience months of debilitating, chronic symptoms—some of which are autoimmune in nature—and we don't understand why. It's possible that the infection alters the immune system and/or damages organs somehow to perpetuate symptoms even though the virus is gone. Put simply, the bug acts like a hit-and-run villain to leave the person vulnerable to other ailments.

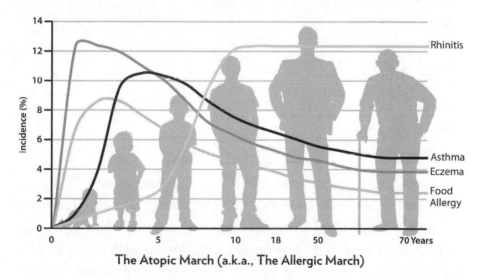

The Atopic March (a.k.a., The Allergic March)

This idea that having one allergic disease (e.g., atopic dermatitis or food allergy) may in turn increase risk of developing subsequent allergic diseases (e.g., allergic rhinitis or asthma) is something that we addressed in earlier discussions of the "allergic march." However, it's important to note that these are not the only conditions that are strongly associated with food allergy. In our recent survey of more than fifty thousand US households, our team assessed the prevalence of a wide variety of immune-mediated chronic conditions. The following table shows how estimated rates of current food allergy prevalence are much higher among US children and adults with these other immune-mediated conditions, compared to the general US population, where 7.6 percent of children (more than five million) and 10.8 percent of adults (more than twenty-six million) are estimated to be food allergic.

PHYSICIAN-DIAGNOSED CONDITIONS . . .	RATES OF FOOD ALLERGY AMONG US CHILDREN	RATES OF FOOD ALLERGY AMONG US ADULTS
Allergic rhinitis	18%	17%
Asthma	20%	21%
Atopic dermatitis/eczema	19%	19%
Eosinophilic esophagitis	32%	37%
FPIES	65%	43%
Insect sting allergy	22%	23%
Latex allergy	49%	29%
Medication allergy	18%	19%
Urticaria/chronic hives	31%	28%

What I want you to remember from this chapter is that all the factors I covered—chiefly an imbalanced microbiome and a dysfunctional immune system—all play into inflammatory pathways. Throughout the rest of the book, we'll see how taming inflammation will be key to gaining control—and preventing—food allergies and intolerances.

Modernity conspires to confuse our old-fashioned, albeit clever body. In the previous chapter, I focused mostly on environmental factors in diet and sanitation. But others are part of the equation, such as stress in general. Modern society dictates we do more all the time, and the resulting psychological stress has a deep impact on our physiology that can, in turn, raise risks for food-related conditions.

You might be surprised to learn that stress can even impact the microbiome in unimaginable ways. Sudden anxiety or being temporarily nervous can be unpleasant, but it's not particularly damaging to the microbiome. Destructive stress, on the other hand, is the unabating kind, which can have more serious effects on the gut and risk for disease. Without going into too much detail, suffice it say that experimental studies show that toxic stress stagnates digestion in the small intestine, which can lead to an overgrowth of bacteria there, which then compromises that delicate intestinal barrier. Unfriendly bacteria are allowed to proliferate, crowding out the beneficial bugs and changing the gut composition—leading to dysbiosis and opening the door to a host of negative effects, the least of which can result in allergic disorders in vulnerable people. Once again, this goes to show the interconnectivity of the human body. Like a giant, complex spiderweb, when you pull one tiny thread, the whole contraption moves. How exactly it moves and how it's damaged depends, metaphorically, on the type of spider, its style of cobweb, and whether the lattice is pulled gently, tugged, or yanked.

To think that stress could be a root cause of these ailments is astonishing, but stress physiology has come a long way in the last several decades. Although the cascade of events that occur in the body when it's under stress has been well defined for a long time, newer research is finally revealing its relationship with diverse conditions not previously tied to stress, allergic diseases and food intolerances among them. Jane will never know how much the stressful year preceding her rheumatoid arthritis diagnosis contributed to the condition, but it likely played a role. Similarly, Lauren's stress load probably bore some of the blame, too, in the progression of her ailments.

Research is currently under way, including my own, to reveal the relationship of stress and anxiety to allergic conditions. We know stress impacts health in so many ways and its impact on allergy is currently being explored. Adults who suddenly and unexpectedly develop food allergies could owe some of their disease onset to stress. They also, as with their children, have witnessed and experienced a revolution in food manufacturing and farming practices. As noted, we have to wonder how modern agricultural practices impact risk for food allergies and intolerances at any age. Does our modern cornucopia of food indulgences ultimately deceive us? That conversation is deserving of its own chapter. . . .

Fearless Facts

→ Food is more than fuel; it's information for the body and may impact how your genes express themselves through epigenetic effects. This helps explain how underlying genetics can influence risk of disease, including the full spectrum of adverse food-related reactions discussed up to this point.

→ The health of your gut's intestinal lining—the single cell layer or barrier between your gut's insides and the rest of your body via your circulation—is extremely important. In addition to being a major player in your immune system, your intestinal microbiome also factors into the strength and function of your intestinal wall. Imbalances in your gut flora that in turn lead to compromises in your intestinal wall, often called leaky gut in layman's terms, may lead to numerous health challenges—from food-related reactions to metabolic disorders and autoimmunity.

→ Chronic psychological stress can "get under the skin" and have major influences on immune function, including allergic disease outcomes. While data are still emerging, systematic efforts to address chronic stressors hold promise for improvement of physical and psychological health—including a variety of allergic disease-related outcomes. (See Chapter 8 for more information, including stress-reduction strategies.)

five

CAUTION: MAY CONTAIN...

A Cornucopia of Confusion

THE NEXT TIME YOU BITE INTO A JUICY CHEESEBURGER OR WATCH SOMEONE else do the same, think about where all of those ingredients came from—the beef, bun, cheese, lettuce, tomato, onions, pickles, sauces, and seasonings. You might picture nine or so "simple" ingredients (maybe you skip the onions and cheese) and imagine a few family-run farms in middle America supplying the delicious makings. You might be surprised to learn that the reality of creating that burger is much more complex and far from simple. The finished entrée reflects a cornucopia of ingredients coming together from a vast assemblage of sources. In fact, if I were to flash a visual that reflects the intricacies of the global food supply chain to arrive at your grub, you'd be dazed, bewildered, maybe impressed. Between primary production and you as the hungry consumer on the receiving end, there's a dizzying array of junctures you'd never guess take place (nor where).

Following the production of a classic cheeseburger is actually a powerful way to visually imagine and mentally grasp this labyrinth. Working with a large quick-service restaurant franchise, researchers at the University of Minnesota mapped the global supply chain of a cheeseburger. They followed the movement of different commodities from the farm through processing to the restaurant, identifying all the ingredients found in this company's cheeseburgers. They included the variety of companies supplying key ingredients, such as vinegar, garlic powder, tomatoes, beef, and wheat gluten. Each cheeseburger included more than fifty ingredients sourced from countries in every continent of the world except Antarctica. Not only is it possible that the ingredients were all sourced from far outside the US, but take any single ingredient, such as the perfectly square "American cheese," and you'll find a long list of components: milk, milk fat, water, cream, sodium citrate, salt, sodium phosphate, sorbic acid, artificial flavor, cheese culture, acetic acid, soy lecithin, enzymes, and starch. And that's just the cheese! You may not even recognize some of these ingredients, and within "artificial flavor" is probably some nifty chemistry. The basic burger is anything but basic. It's a modern marvel.

Take a moment to think about all the marvels of the modern world, in fact, from computer technology and transportation to rapid access to goods and services that make life exceedingly easier. In the food realm, we can walk into a grocery store and buy any food we want, even when certain items are not in season or were cultivated and packaged thousands of miles—sometimes oceans—away. Some of us don't even have to bother physically going to a brick-and-mortar store anymore; we can order online and have our purchases delivered to our doorstep within hours.

Now, let's reverse this picture. Imagine time-traveling back to the era of hunter-gatherers and toting a bag or two of your typical groceries with you (bring the burger too). Would your ancestors recognize your daily sustenance? They may identify with the eggs, fruits, and vegetables (though they'd probably be amazed at having so much variety all at once), but they'd be confused by a lot of your staples. The neatly layered burger with all its fixings bookended by the buns and that fits so well in the hands would be particularly interesting to them. Assuming they could read nutrition labels, your ancestors would likely stumble over many ingredients and wonder at the snazzy packaging. A vast majority of your groceries may be totally foreign and unrecognizable.

I am asked often about modern food manufacturing and the global supply chain in the context of food allergies. Food manufacturing and farming practices have transformed a lot over the past several decades. How much have some of these changes affected the rise in allergies? What does it mean for our body when we consume products that have been altered from their natural state? (And, I should interject that the word "natural" is often misunderstood.) What about hidden additives, fish farmed in warehouse tanks, and genetically modified organisms (GMOs)? Or are some of the criticisms often launched at the food industry overly hyped as is the organic movement? Is the Western diet heavy in ultraprocessed grub to blame? Why is food allergen management during production so difficult? Is there hope we can rely on the industry to protect us?

These are questions with complex answers, and much still remains unknown, but you'd be surprised by the fact our foods today are incredibly sterile—much more so than what people ate hundreds of years ago. And yes, there is hope for a safer food industry. Regulations in farming practices and food manufacturing in general have made our supplies safe for the most part. Sure, there will always be some unsavory operators and corner-cutting, as in any industry, but overall, modern food supplies are remarkably robust and salubrious. What's challenging, however, is how foods get labeled and how we account for potential allergens.

As part of a family that needs to read labels carefully to avoid foods due to allergies, it is my goal to stand up for all families with food conditions and help demand better labeling and process. After speaking at a conference on the importance of this, many food industry representatives started telling me their obstacles. One I remember clearly stated, "How do we know that the same burlap bag that is used to collect cocoa is not used to collect peanuts when it is happening on another continent from which these ingredients are sourced?" A fair question.

In 2017, my colleagues and I wrote a paper that reviewed perspectives from within the food industry, especially with regard to the challenges that manufacturers commonly confront while trying to keep their food-allergic customers safe. We need to find better ways to do this together as one of the biggest expenses reported by industry was recalls. Those findings will be highlighted here with an important lesson: the food industry has shifted not just how we eat but what we eat—sometimes for better, other times for worse. As I've already implied, food production is more efficient and available than ever before; we can eat spring greens in autumn, buy winter squash in summer, and basically eat whatever we want whenever we want due to a massive global distribution network for foods and food products. Moreover, we can manufacture foods in ways that can feed more people in our ever-expanding population. This is good news, because food insecurity remains a global scourge with more than 800 million people living every day with hunger or no reliable access to a sufficient quantity of affordable, nutritious food.

In this chapter, we're going to take a quick tour of the food industry and further address the question as to why certain migration patterns among people offer clues to the food allergy epidemic. Between the marvels of modern food production to mobility patterns around the world, the spectrum of adverse food reactions only grows more complex and expansive. To be sure, this is far from a "bash the food industry" diatribe. The data for making a strong case against the modern food industry are still in their infancy and, in many ways, weak (despite the media scrutiny they often receive). Clearly, the food industry offers an ever-expanding variety of food, prepared in increasingly novel ways. From my perspective, what's most important is to work together to ensure appropriate regulations are in place to advise and protect consumers with food allergies, intolerances, and other food-related conditions.

FROM FARM TO TABLE?

The food supply chain from production to consumption is like a maze whose cipher to get through it resembles a treasure map. Everyone eats, so no one escapes relying on food systems unless one is totally self-sufficient and "off the grid," as they say. Food systems are diverse, elaborate, and dynamic. They involve everything from subsistence farming to multinational food companies and are at the mercy of multiple forces—the weather, demographics, economics, technological advances, entrepreneurism, and consumer preferences. Packaged foods are made and assembled primarily in commercial food processing facilities, which range from very large corporations that may make dozens of different products within a single facility to very small businesses that tend to make a narrower range of products but also often share facilities with other small producers. Packaged foods can also be made in restaurants, retail grocery stores, and other retail outlets. The increasing demand for "ready-to-eat" foods has sparked the growth of quick-service restaurants and fully cooked, frozen dishes that only require reheating. This reflects yet another hallway in the vast labyrinth that further expands the supply chain and complicates the picture.

In addition, food processing equipment is frequently shared to make different products. Although many of us like to aim for whole, unprocessed foods and like to think we're "eating directly from nature," it's virtually impossible to have a diet that's not part of the global food supply and processing system to some degree. Mind you, processing encompasses a wide spectrum—from something as simple as picking a fruit from the vine to be packaged for the local farmers' market to the sophisticated practices that give us cereal, bread, cheese, and candy. Adding to the complexity is the fact that a packaged food may contain several dozen ingredients procured from a range of suppliers who themselves probably also have upstream suppliers. The movement of food and its ingredients includes animals and animal products, plants and plant products, minerals, and vitamins. The farms and other suppliers that are sources of these ingredients (e.g., oceans, mines) are also often diversified and often share harvesting and planting equipment, transportation vehicles, and storage facilities. We can't forget about all the behind-the-scenes aspects we don't think about—the agricultural inputs, such as feed, fertilizer, vaccines, and pharmaceuticals.

The Lingo of Food Label Language

As you can guess, allergens can enter foods from many sources along the food chain, intentionally or unintentionally, through cross-contact in farms, storage, distribution and manufacturing facilities, food service establishments, or the home. The food industry, of course, wishes to prevent the possibility that someone with a food allergy will experience an adverse reaction after eating a packaged food product. In reality, achieving this goal at all times is not easy, but the manufacturers are doing their best and investing a lot of money into making their products as safe as possible.

From the food industry perspective, three general approaches are used to minimize the risk of a reaction from an allergenic food: (1) eliminate potential allergens or specific allergens from products; (2) list the allergen on the product label as an ingredient, when it is intentionally added as such; and (3) implement strict allergen control plans to minimize allergen contamination and use advisory labels (e.g., *May contain . . .*) to inform people about the risk when necessary.

Clearly, all of us rely on food manufacturers to reliably track and declare the presence of food allergens in products. Over the past two decades, the food industry has increasingly adopted allergen control approaches in its processing facilities. Nearly all major food manufacturers that supply the American market (92 percent) produced food products containing one or more of the top nine allergenic foods recognized by the FDA. The FDA has established "Good Manufacturing Practices," which outline specific requirements for the production of processed foods. These include tracing the movement of raw materials through the supply chain, handling of materials during processing, and appropriate labeling of final food products.

In 2004, the FDA enacted the Food Allergen Labeling and Consumer Protection Act (FALCPA). The FALCPA applies to the labeling of foods regulated by the FDA, which includes all foods except poultry, most meats, certain egg products, and most alcoholic beverages (these are regulated by other federal agencies). The FALCPA requires that food labels clearly identify the food source names of any ingredients that are "major food allergens" or contain any protein derived from a "major food allergen," which includes the following nine common allergens: milk, eggs, fish (e.g., bass, flounder, cod), crustacean shellfish (e.g., crab, lobster, shrimp), tree nuts (e.g., almonds, walnuts, pecans), peanuts, wheat, soybeans, and, as of 2021, sesame. The FDA exempts highly refined oils, such as peanut and soybean oil, from being labeled as an allergen, as they are usually safe for people with soy allergies (although some companies do still provide source labeling).

Note that as I write this, molluscan shellfish—such as oysters, clams, mussels, or scallops—are not required to be labeled as a major allergen. Sesame will start to be labeled as a major allergen in 2023. For years, my colleague Christopher Warren, PhD, has led our team's efforts to help the US Department of Health and Human Services (HHS)—which oversees the FDA, CDC, and NIH—and other stakeholders understand the magnitude of the food allergy epidemic, so that appropriate public health policies can be crafted and implemented. Together, through numerous national surveys, we have helped US policymakers understand the extent to which sesame seed, mollusks, and other lesser-known food allergens currently affect US children and adults. For example, two recent studies found that roughly half of US children and adults with crustacean shellfish allergy are also allergic to mollusks. We published another study in 2019 in response to a request from the FDA for data about the frequency and severity of sesame seed allergy, which highlighted that sesame seed allergy and severe allergic reactions were more common than previously acknowledged in the US. Each of these studies raises concern about areas where current allergen labeling laws can potentially be improved to better protect the growing number of US children and adults living with food allergy.

Currently under FALCPA, US law requires that food labels identify the food source names of all major food allergens used to make the food. This requirement is met if the common or usual name of an ingredient (e.g., buttermilk) that is a major food allergen already identifies that allergen's food source name (in this example, milk). Otherwise, the allergen's food source name must be declared at least once on the food label in one of two ways.

The first way is to name the food source of a major food allergen in parentheses following the name of the ingredient. Examples: "lecithin (soy)," "flour (wheat)," and "whey (milk)." The other way is to call out the potentially problematic ingredients immediately after or next to the entire list of ingredients in a "contains" statement. For example: "Contains wheat, milk, and soy." We've all gotten used to seeing these labels on foods, but they don't always tell the whole story. I'll be going into more specific details about how to read a label in the next part, but I want to give you a primer here.

The FALCPA's labeling requirements do not apply to the potential or unintentional presence of major food allergens in foods resulting from "cross-contact" situations during manufacturing. In the context of food allergens, cross-contact occurs when a residue or trace amount of an allergenic food becomes incorporated into another food not intended to contain it; simply put, it's the unintentional introduction of allergen residues into a product that does not contain them as ingredients. FDA guidance for the food industry states that food allergen advisory statements, such as "may contain [allergen]" or "produced in a facility that also uses [allergen]" should not be used as a substitute for adhering to current Good Manufacturing Practices and must be truthful and not misleading. These guidelines were updated in 2011 through the passage of the Food Safety Modernization Act (FSMA), which identifies food allergen cross-contact as one of the key hazards that needs to be evaluated.

When allergens have been identified as a hazard, the food manufacturing facilities are required under FSMA to establish elaborate preventive allergen control measures.

A big caveat: Current guidelines do not establish specific requirements for allergen control during the *manufacturing* process. Although efforts are typically made to segregate foods containing major allergens during manufacturing, cross-contact may occur due to processing on shared equipment, mishandling during packaging, or the use of raw ingredients coming in unanalyzed from all parts of the world and difficulty of cleaning equipment. Consequently, manufacturers routinely develop and implement independent allergen control plans to minimize the risk of product contact with food allergen contaminants and prevent recall events due to undeclared allergens. These plans typically specify practices for the safe handling and storage of raw materials, employee training, facility and equipment design, cleaning procedures, and production scheduling.

In addition, companies may use precautionary allergen labeling (PAL) on packaging to label products for which there is a risk of cross-contact with food allergens during production. But, unfortunately, such measures remain *voluntary* and *unregulated*, and such labeling currently presents us all with considerable challenges due to its inconsistent use. Although these labels are not legally required, *almost half of consumers think they are*. What's more, the meaning of these labels ("may contain") can be confusing for consumers. There are many variations of wording used in these labels, but the different wording does not indicate the likelihood or the potential amount of the allergen. My own study of labels found over twenty-five different types of wording for precautionary allergen labels, such as these examples:

"May contain traces of nuts"
"Processed in a facility that also processes peanuts"
"Manufactured on equipment that also processes peanuts"
"Not suitable for people with peanut allergy"

"Good manufacturing practices used to segregate ingredients
in a facility that also processes peanuts."

People can be left asking questions: What's the chance it contains
an allergenic ingredient? And if it does, how much? Enough to cause a
reaction? More than half of consumers—53 percent—say that current
labeling practices pose a significant problem that interferes with their
daily lives. Labeling in the food industry is indeed not perfect and begs
to be revolutionized. I have plenty of stories from patients whose allergic reactions came from unexpected allergen cross-contact when they
thought they'd done everything right to prevent such an event. In our
world where it is often difficult to avoid PAL and risks are taken, nearly
a quarter of people in our survey said they had experienced a reaction
from a food with a PAL label on it.

Future regulations will only clean up the industry more so and give
people greater peace of mind. I speak on this topic routinely in both lay
and professional circles, including food industry summits, to keep people
informed about labeling practices and galvanize efforts to reform policies
based on some of my own research. One exciting development in this
area is the recent passage of the Food Allergy Safety, Treatment, Education, and Research (FASTER) Act that President Biden signed into law in
2021. The stated aim of this bill is: "To improve the health and safety of
Americans living with food allergies and related disorders, including potentially life-threatening anaphylaxis, food protein-induced enterocolitis
syndrome, and eosinophilic gastrointestinal diseases, and for other purposes." One of the key provisions of this bill updated FALCPA to protect the nearly 1.6 million Americans allergic to sesame and require the
mandatory labeling of sesame-containing foods, while another directs
the secretary of Health and Human Services (HHS) to issue a report on
scientific opportunities in food allergy research that examines prevention, treatment, and new cures. In addition, the legislation establishes a
risk-based scientific process and framework for establishing additional
allergens covered by the Federal Food, Drug, and Cosmetic Act.

For years, our team's national food allergy surveys have been a leading source of information about the prevalence and severity of food allergies in the US. With the recent passage of the FASTER Act, we have the opportunity to work alongside experts from the CDC to make the most accurate possible estimates of the public heath burden of food allergies in the US. I admit, it has been so exciting and inspiring to see Congress express such near-unanimous enthusiasm for food allergy research and affected patients through its bipartisan support of the FASTER Act.

In 2020, my team published a study that sought to understand food allergy stakeholders' preferences for precautionary allergen labeling. We asked them about their understanding of labeling policies, current shopping habits, how they generally feel about the use of precautionary allergen labeling (PAL), and what language, placement, and format would help them feel more comfortable when shopping for packaged foods. After analyzing data from over three thousand respondents nationwide, we found some consistently shocking results. About 1 in 4 respondents reported experiencing an allergic reaction from a product containing a PAL statement. Only about a quarter of respondents were aware that precautionary allergen labeling is only voluntarily placed by the manufacturers, and many believed PAL wording ("may contain," "manufactured in a facility," etc.) was placed depending on the amount of allergen used in the products. Moreover, we found that participants were shopping for certain PALs wordings more than others, despite the fact that no single phrase is regulated.

Finally, when it came to choosing a phrase that they'd like to see moving forward, the majority chose the label "not suitable for," which indicates that they'd really like a clear phrase that shows them whether the food is safe for them. The next favorite was "may contain." This is well-known wording and is the recommended labeling in Canada. Having just this without the many other options may decrease confusion on their meanings. People want clear messaging; they do not want to interpret the meaning and the foods' potential safety. We are working with scientists and industry to see how we can make this happen. The majority of respondents—especially those with multiple food allergies—said they'd feel more confident about buying foods with PAL if there was a declarative statement on products designating the manufacturers use an allergen-free *facility* (with specific allergens listed) or a declarative statement on products designating the manufacturers use an allergen free *line* (with specific allergens listed). There is also a clear desire for threshold amounts for PAL. This is something many researchers are working on, as well as the Food Allergy Research and Resource Program (FARRP). In an ideal world, it would be nice to know your individual threshold of allergen (what can your body tolerate without reacting) and know the allergen threshold in a food product with a PAL statement. This is what many organizations and scientists are striving for. We will need to work on policy with insurance companies to make sure that threshold testing can be covered along with access to safe allergen-free foods.

Also, as we continue to work on this, I do want to appreciate the many small companies that have grown from individual passion to help keep people safe and clearly keep allergens out of their products. I also commend the companies that help curate the lists of trusted brands in this area and in Appendix B you will find lists of resources that keeps growing every day.

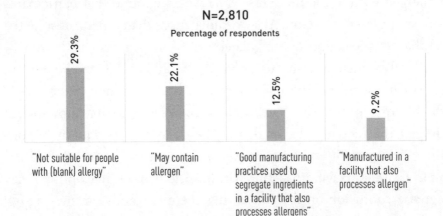

N=2,810

Percentage of respondents

29.3%	22.1%	12.5%	9.2%
"Not suitable for people with (blank) allergy"	"May contain allergen"	"Good manufacturing practices used to segregate ingredients in a facility that also processes allergens"	"Manufactured in a facility that also processes allergen"

All of these results make it abundantly clear that more education is needed for food allergy families to make safe decisions while grocery shopping, and more work is done to find consistent phrasing to help them along the way. We've used these data to help both manufacturers and the FDA govern appropriate policies around PAL, and although it's a work in progress, it's integral to keeping anyone with food allergy safe.

Organic Foods, GMOs, and Allergens

Foods labeled organic are all the rage today. At the same time, there's a growing movement against foods made with genetically modified organisms (GMO). But confusion abounds about what these terms actually mean and how much of an impact they are having in the risk for allergies. When you shop in a grocery store, you're likely to encounter the word "organic" everywhere but not so much "GMO" (you'll come across more "GMO-free" labels than "Made with GMO"). You might think that food grown organically would be free of allergens, but this is a misconception. You might also think that GMO is meticulously labeled for you to see, but it's not. Although the industry itself is regulated for production, standardized labeling has yet to fully catch up.

Organic foods may be free of harmful pesticides, but they aren't free of the proteins that cause allergic reactions. People tend to equate the word "organic" or "natural" with "healthy" and, in turn, "safe." But organic or natural does not mean allergen-free (or safe for that matter; many poisons, such as anthrax and arsenic, are natural and organic!). The following chart represents the USDA requirements set forth for organic foods and shows differences between organic and natural. While there are benefits of organic and natural food, in some cases, remember that neither guarantee allergy-safe, and organic foods sometimes come at an additional financial cost.

People are readily confused by organic labeling, so let's clarify. The USDA Organic Seal indicates that a food was produced without synthetic pesticides, genetically modified organisms (GMOs), or fertilizers

USDA Organic vs. Natural

	ORGANIC	NATURAL
Toxic persistent pesticides	not allowed	allowed
GMOs	not allowed	allowed
Antibiotics	not allowed	allowed
Growth hormones	not allowed	allowed
Sludge and irradiation	not allowed	allowed
Animal welfare requirements	yes	no
Cows required to be on pasture for pasture season	yes	no
Lower levels of environmental pollution	yes	not necessarily
Audit trail from farm to table	yes	no
Certification required, including inspections	yes	no
Legal restrictions on allowable materials	yes	no

made from petroleum (e.g., ammonium nitrate, superphosphate, and potassium sulfate). When it comes to organic meats and dairy products, the seal bears even more weight: it also means that the meats or dairy products are from animals that are fed organic feed and forage, are not treated with antibiotics or hormones, and are raised in living conditions that accommodate their natural behaviors, such as grazing. Only foods made with 100 percent organic ingredients can indicate that on the label. If a food was made with at least 95 percent organic ingredients, then it can say just the word "organic." Products that say "Made with organic ingredients" were created with a minimum of 70 percent organic ingredients, with restrictions on the remaining 30 percent, including no GMOs.

My whole point in bringing these definitions up is to underscore an important lesson: the word "organic" has various definitions depending on where it's applied, and organic does not equate with allergen-free. Someone with an oral allergy to kiwifruit, for example, can have a reaction to both the conventionally grown and organic varieties. A question that many people with food allergies ask, however, is whether animal feed—organic or not—that contains allergens can trickle down into the products made from those animals. For example, if chickens are given soy and/or peanut proteins in their feed, do the eggs and meat produced from them also contain those problematic proteins? Turns out that studies so far show that, no, those allergens in the feed do not transfer to their meat and eggs.

Now, those GMOs. I field lots of questions about the relationship between GMO foods and allergies. But before we address those concerns, let's first get some general definitions out of the way. What does GMO mean?

GMOs are plants or animals that have been genetically engineered with DNA from other living things, including bacteria, viruses, plants, and animals. The genetic combinations that result do not happen naturally in the wild or in traditional crossbreeding. This is the heart of the controversy—that these are "unnatural." GMO foods are often created to fight pests that can destroy crops, or to cultivate crops with certain desired characteristics. The reason a lot of Hawaiian papayas are GMO, for example, is that the ring spot virus decimated nearly half of the state's papaya crop in the 1990s. In 1998, scientists developed a genetically engineered version of the papaya called the Rainbow papaya, which is resistant to the virus. Now more than 70 percent of the papayas grown in Hawaii are GMO. Many crops, in fact, have been engineered to create a product that is more nutritious or resistant to disease.

It helps to think of GMOs as divided into three broad categories. The first category includes foods engineered to produce a nutrient that they would not otherwise contain. They are biofortified using GMO (to be clear, "biofortified" can include genetic modification but also covers other, non-GMO methods for improving the nutritional quality of crops). For example, to combat vitamin A deficiency in many parts of the world where malnutrition and food insecurity are endemic, scientists have leveraged GMO to turn a form of normal white rice into a yellow-colored rice that provides beta-carotene, a precursor of vitamin A.

Fortified Golden Rice remains hotly debated and controversial and has yet to be accepted worldwide and made commercially available but it's a prime example of how GMO could potentially address health problems and save lives. Vitamin A deficiency may not be an issue in the Western world, but it kills up to two million people and causes blindness in more than half a million children worldwide each year.

The second category includes crops engineered to be resistant to some pathogens, such as the case with Hawaiian papaya. But this kind of engineering can result in allergenic proteins from these modified genes mistakenly introduced into the food supply. But again, my hope is these GMOs are well studied and tightly regulated. Also note that because food allergens are almost exclusively proteins, it is possible to study the amino acid sequence of emerging GMO protein candidates and comparing their amino acid sequences to those of known food allergens. This is one way to help understand which GMOs may be most likely to have allergenic properties. In the future, we may be able to cultivate plants, for instance, that lack the most problematic proteins.

Finally, the third broad category includes crops designed to be resistant to one or more chemical pesticides and weed killers. This is the category that gives GMOs a bad name. The farming practices that are involved with this type of GMO have raised concerns among environmentalists and some doctors due to the level of agrochemicals that can be used. Seeds planted in this category are genetically modified to be resistant to a chemical's effects, but it means farmers can use those chemicals, one of which—glyphosate—has gained notoriety for its potential carcinogenic attributes (in 2017, California became the first state in the nation to issue a warning on glyphosate by adding the chemical to the state's Proposition 65 list of chemicals and substances known to cause cancer). The increasing use of herbicides means that GMO and conventionally farmed crops are almost invariably contaminated with herbicides and other agrochemicals. Corn and soy are the top two GMO crops in the United States, followed closely by canola and sugar beets; these ingredients are frequently used in processed foods. In fact, it has been estimated that GMOs are in as much as 80 percent of con ventional processed foods (though you may not know it when you eat those processed foods due to lack of labeling). According to the FDA, scientists developing GMOs run tests to make sure allergens are not transferred from one food to another. And again, I should reiterate that research shows that GMO foods are no more likely to cause allergies than non-GMOs.

Most GMO crops are not directly consumed by humans. GMO corn is used in animal feed and high-fructose corn syrup, and GMO soy makes soybean and vegetable oils, soy protein, and more heavily processed soy, such as lecithin, and flavorings that land in a trove of processed products. If you are a conventional meat, egg, or dairy eater, the animals those foods come from are eating lots of GMO corn and soy. Even strict vegetarians and vegans may not escape GMOs; if they eat conventional veggie burgers and soy dogs, they are likely made with GMO soy.

We know that GMO products do not appear to be more allergenic than their conventional counterparts from IgE-binding studies (to be sure, if you're allergic to certain fruits and vegetables, that doesn't mean GMO versions are allergen free). The technology used for making GMO crops does not necessarily make us more vulnerable than conventional breeding. Genetically modified crops undergo rigorous assessment for food, feed, and environmental safety before commercialization. When assessing for allergenic potential, several questions are addressed, such as the source and sequence of a new gene introduced to the crop that codes for proteins, how abundant the newly expressed protein is in the food, and whether it's resistant to digestive acids.

Since GMO market approval is under strict regulation, we should probably be more concerned about contamination from unauthorized GMOs than about allergies to common GMO foods. You may remember, for instance, a recall of hard taco shells in the early 2000s that included varieties used by Taco Bell. The GMO corn involved contained a specially engineered protein that makes the corn resistant to insects, but it was not supposed to be consumed by humans because it had not passed one test needed for full approval for humans. The corn had only been approved for animal feed but somehow leaked into the food supply, resulting in significant disruption of the supply. Although there were concerns that the GMO corn contained a potential human allergen, there was no evidence that anyone had an allergic reaction. Since this incident, which was the first-ever recall of a genetically modified food, regulations governing GMOs have gotten stricter, to the point we can have pretty good faith in most GMO products when they are carefully made with oversight.

According to the US Department of Agriculture (USDA): The use of genetic engineering, or genetically modified organisms (GMOs), is prohibited in organic products. This means an organic farmer can't plant GMO seeds, an organic cow can't eat GMO alfalfa or corn, and an organic soup producer can't use any GMO ingredients. To meet the USDA organic regulations, farmers and processors must show they aren't using GMOs and that they are protecting their products from contact with prohibited substances, such as GMOs, from farm to table. Common foods that are made with GMO ingredients or are derived from GMO-exposed animals include:

Premade soups

Frozen meals

Nondairy soy milk products (e.g., soy milk,
    soy formula, soy ice cream, soy creamer)

Juice drinks and soda

Cereals

Chips

Vegetable oils

Tofu

Conventional meat and dairy

Some meat substitutes

Spices and seasoning mixes

Soft drinks and fruit juice

Dried fruit

Because GMO foods are relatively new to the scene, we need more research to truly understand their impact on our health, allergies, and intolerances. We also need more clear labeling laws to know where GMO foods are found. Transparency is important, and for people with food allergies nothing could be more vital to living free from constant food fear. As any individual with food-related conditions will tell you, especially someone with multiple food allergies, taking a bite out of something that you don't know what it contains can be frightening. And nothing could be more anxiety-stirring than hidden food allergens that either escape proper labeling or are delivered to you outside of their original packaging and labeling, as happens in restaurants and cafeterias.

HIDDEN FOOD ALLERGENS

Although we often think about modern farming practices causing unwanted ingredients in our food supply, we fail to realize that they can also render foods *missing* certain ingredients our bodies expect. Many plants contain fewer nutrients than they used to; because of soil depletion, crops grown decades ago were much richer in vitamins and minerals than the varieties most of us get today. A study by Donald Davis and his team of researchers from the University of Texas (UT) at Austin's Department of Chemistry and Biochemistry first sounded the alarm in 2004 in the *Journal of the American College of Nutrition* and which reached mainstream headline news. They reviewed US Department of Agriculture nutritional data from both 1950 and 1999 for forty-three different vegetables and fruits, finding "statistically reliable declines" in the amount of protein, calcium, phosphorus, iron, riboflavin (vitamin B_2) and vitamin C over the past half century. Seven other nutrients they looked at showed no change. Davis and his colleagues explained the declining nutritional content—the "dilution effect"—of certain nutrients by way of agricultural practices designed to improve traits (size, growth rate, pest resistance) other than nutrition. Other studies I've read suggest that different breeding techniques also can change how plants absorb nutrients from the soil; however, this is an active area of investigation and the implications of these findings for human health and nutrition remain unclear.

I also want to make clear that more recent studies have challenged the extent of the nutrient declines summarized in the previous paragraph and argue that changes in mineral concentrations, for instance, are "within natural variation ranges and are not nutritionally significant," and that we're not about to lose out on our daily recommended serving of nutrients when we eat well. The debate has also entered the organic arena where studies show that organic foods are oversold as being more nutritious. Again, I expect these debates to continue. One thing we all can agree on is that food processing in general can change the composition of foods our body was once used to and shift how they are accepted by the body (kale chips do not nourish the body the same way as a fresh kale salad does). When you turn whole grains into refined products, for instance, you lose the fiber that's so important for health—including that of the microbiome.

Earlier I compared the diets of our ancestors to the pleasures of modern food choices. That conversation does not mean we all should be on a Paleo, or "caveman," diet. Although our ancestors ate many different foods, it was almost always the same array of foods year after year and lifetime after lifetime. Their body was a well-oiled machine. Today, our eating behaviors are vastly different, a result, as I've been detailing, of both food manufacturing and farming practices as well as changes in access to certain foods.

Avoiding problematic foods, such as eggs or dairy, might seem simple enough at first, but it can be a minefield if you eat out a lot. Here are the most common ways the top five food allergens can hide in everyday foods (note that the following lists are partial—for more comprehensive lists and sublists, go to www.FoodAllergy.org):

Peanuts: Foods that may contain peanuts and should be avoided by those suffering from a peanut allergy include salad dressings, chocolate candy bars, Asian-style dipping sauces, nougat, ice cream, egg and spring rolls, chili, energy bars, graham cracker crust, and marzipan (among many other items—see Chapter 9). Note that how peanuts are harvested and processed can affect the allergenic properties of their proteins. Boiled peanuts, for example, can cause a weaker allergic reaction or no reaction at all in some people (roasted peanuts are more allergenic). This is an active area of research.

Eggs: The whites of the egg contain the allergy-causing proteins. Egg protein can often be hidden in such foods as baked goods, mayonnaise, egg substitute, egg pasta (macaroni/lasagne), egg noodles, artificial crabmeat, and meringues. Note that yolks always contain residues of egg white proteins, so egg white–allergic people are at risk if they try to eat egg yolk ingredients.

Milk and milk-containing food: As I've already explained, an allergy to milk is different from being lactose intolerant because it involves the immune system, which reacts adversely to a protein in the milk. Avoiding milk products is not as easy as you might expect because they can still be found in such foods as coffee creamers, custards, gravies, and peanut butter, all of which may use some form of milk solids. They can wind up in many unsuspecting places, such as canned tuna, granola mixes, and crackers. Casein and caseinates, for example, are proteins in milk that can be found in such products as canned tuna fish, dental chewing gums, and even breath mints. Milk proteins in general can be disguised by any number of ingredients: butter, cheese, whipped cream, ghee, hydrolysates, whey . . . to name just a few. Words like natural flavoring, flavoring, caramel flavoring, high protein flour, rice cheese, and soy cheese, and even *nondairy* or *pareve* could also be code for foods that contain milk proteins. As a reminder, if any of these food ingredients intentionally contain milk, then they must be labeled (FALCPA). They may contain residues unintentionally, of course.

Wheat: Avoiding wheat is tough because it finds its way into so many products that use it as a binding or thickening agent. Remember: This is not the same as gluten intolerance in celiac disease or a gluten sensitivity, but can be very severe in some cases. Foods to avoid that may contain wheat include cereal and cereal bars, couscous, pasta/noodles, bread/bread crumbs, bulgur, spelt, ice cream with cookie dough, ready-made burgers, beer, and soy sauce. In some cases, inhaling wheat flour can also be problematic.

Soy: Soybeans are often used in most processed foods, which means it is hidden in a large range of foods. These are the most common foods where it is found: miso, cereal, baked goods, crackers, prepared meats (e.g., sausage and lunch meats), margarine, shortening, some peanut butters, canned tuna, canned soups (and it is the main ingredient in tofu and tempeh). It can also hide in vegetable broth, vegetable oil, sauces, "natural flavorings," and ingredients that go by their food-tech chemical names: hydrolyzed vegetable protein, textured vegetable protein, lecithin, monodiglyceride, and monosodium glutamate (MSG). By some estimates, soy is found in an estimated 60 percent of processed foods. Note that soy oil (unless cold pressed or expeller pressed) and soy lecithin are typically safe for those with soy allergy.

Sesame: Although sesame seeds are often visible on certain foods or dishes, especially Asian and Middle Eastern fare, including tahini and halvah, sesame—and sesame oil—can be hidden within popular foods where you wouldn't expect them to be, such as in bread products. And while sesame doesn't make the top eight for food allergens, it's the ninth culprit and may not be as clearly labeled as the top eight. Sesame allergies may not receive as much publicity as peanut allergies, but the reactions can be just as serious. Uncommon sources of this allergen: baked goods (bagels, breadsticks, hamburger buns, and rolls), bread crumbs, cereals (e.g., granola and muesli), chips (bagel chips, pita chips, and tortilla chips), and crackers (melba toast). Other seeds can also be problematic for a minority of people and can hide in various foods. These include flax, hemp, sunflower, and poppy seeds.

Food Additives and "Agents"

We also cannot neglect adverse reactions that are not classified as food allergy but do indeed take up space on the spectrum of adverse food reactions and often contribute to masqueraders. These include two big buckets of potential culprits my colleague, Dr. Sami Bahna, chief of Allergy/Immunology at Louisiana State University School of Medicine, has discussed and published on: food additives, which encompass reactions to food preservatives, flavoring agents, dyes, emulsifiers, thickeners, stabilizers, or sweeteners (and those additives can hide behind unintelligible names you're not familiar with unless you're a food chemist); and food "agents," which means they are naturally occurring ingredients in foods and not additives. Let's take each of these in turn:

Food additives: Although food additives have been used for thousands of years, in the modern era we have an abundance of more natural and artificial substances than ever before. According to the FDA, there are almost four thousand food additives (so listing them here is beyond the scope of this book). Reactions to additives are rare, but they do happen.

Sulfites are the more common culprits to these reactions. Sulfites are used as preservatives to reduce spoilage, act as antioxidants, and prevent fruits and vegetables from browning prematurely. People with reactions to sulfites can experience mild symptoms, such as a rash, or more serious reactions from worsening asthma to anaphylaxis. Case reports of people reacting to dyes, such as carmine (commonly used for red food coloring) and saffron and annatto (both used for yellow food coloring) have also been reported and implicated in IgE-mediated food allergies. When a patient complains of reactions to commercially prepared foods but has no problem consuming similar homemade foods, my first instinct is to question food additives that could be causing the problem—not the foods themselves.

Food agents: Naturally occurring chemicals in many foods can cause problems in people sensitive to these substances. They may lack an enzyme to properly digest these substances or simply have a digestive system that, possibly due to underlying genetics, processes certain foods differently. Here are some common examples of substances that leave people intolerant:

- Vasoactive amines, such as tyramine, serotonin, and histamine (e.g., in cheeses, processed meats, bananas, pineapple, avocados, citrus fruit, some fermented fish, and sauerkraut). Note that because amines can act directly on small blood vessels to expand their capacity (hence, "vasoactive"), they are likely culprits behind migraines, flushing, and nasal congestion in sensitive people.
- Tryptamine (e.g., in tomato and plum)
- Phenylethylamine (e.g., in chocolate)
- Caffeine (e.g., in coffee, tea, and soft drinks)
- Theobromine and theophylline (e.g., in chocolate and tea)
- Glycoside alkaloid solanine (e.g., in potato)
- Salicylates (found in a wide variety of herbs, spices, fruit, and vegetables)

Besides additives and agents making their mark on the spectrum of adverse food reactions, foodborne toxins can cause adverse food reactions but do not qualify as being allergies—they, too, are masqueraders. These include toxins from bacteria, fungi, and fish—notably, scromboid poisoning in tuna and mackerel; ciguatera toxin poisoning from mackerel, snapper, and barracuda; and saxitoxin from shellfish. Pathogens, such as salmonella, *C. botulinum*, *E. coli*, and listeria in contaminated food that lead to classic food-borne illnesses, also belong to this category. Anyone who has experienced food poisoning knows that the illness can cause severe gastrointestinal distress and sometimes neurological symptoms, but the immune system is not triggered in a life-threatening way.

Finally, accidental contaminants from heavy metals, such as lead, mercury, and copper, arsenic in rice and rice-based foods, pesticides, antibiotics, and dust/storage mites have been reported to cause gastrointestinal symptoms that qualify as an intolerance—a masquerader.

Food Fraud Alert

Reports of food fraud, defined as "the deliberate adulteration, substitution, tampering or misrepresentation of food" is a growing problem worldwide as a result of our complex global food supply chain. Fraud can occur in the raw material, in an ingredient, in the final product, or in the food's packaging. It costs the food industry tens of billions annually. Examples include free-range eggs from caged hens, meat from undeclared sources (e.g., beef burgers containing horsemeat, as happened in the UK and Ireland in 2013), farmed Atlantic salmon sold as wild Pacific king salmon, and the old switcheroo whereby a restaurant owner swaps out say, almond powder, for a cheaper ground nut mix containing peanuts in a sauce so as to save cost. Such a substitution can have devastating consequences if it is not disclosed. Food fraud can also occur when a product contains unsuspecting ingredients: olive oil that has sesame or walnut oil in it; honey that includes corn syrup; saffron spice that is anything but—it's a blend of marigold flowers, turmeric, and grass dyed red to play the part.

Food fraud is a problem for everyone aside from the food allergy epidemic, but for those who do need to be careful about what they eat and know exactly what they are consuming, food fraud adds yet another layer of complexity and potential danger. Not only does fraudulently labeled food undermine companies working legitimately, but foods that contain unlisted or impure ingredients can impact allergies. What's more, ingredients that have been banned can render foods non-compliant with regulations.

Since the thirteenth century during the reign of King John, England has had food fraud laws against diluting wine with water, adding ash to pepper, and packing flour with chalk. Food fraud and adulteration were first addressed in the US by food laws as far back as 1784. In the nineteenth century, the FDA began protecting consumers from snake oil salesmen and other charlatans that preyed on the susceptible public with their alchemy-spiked tonics and elixirs. To help counter this now, the FDA has several hundred agents deployed worldwide as part of its chemical investigations division to investigate food fraud.

Luckily, most food frauds do not result in serious harm, but reports in the past few years show remarkable widespread seafood fraud in particular in the US—even in the finest restaurants. In an alarming study out of UCLA in 2017, the headline said it all: "Bait and Switch . . . Whether to turn a profit or skirt environmental regulations, half the time what's on the menu at L.A. sushi restaurants differs from what's on your plate." When researchers checked the DNA of fish ordered at twenty-six Los Angeles sushi restaurants from 2012 through 2015, they found that 47 percent of sushi was mislabeled. According to the press release announcing the discovery: "The good news is that sushi represented as tuna was almost always tuna. Salmon was mislabeled only about one in 10 times. But out of 43 orders of halibut and 32 orders of red snapper, DNA tests showed the researchers were always served a different kind of fish. A one-year sampling of high-end grocery stores found similar mislabeling rates, suggesting the bait-and-switch may occur earlier in the supply chain than the point of sale to consumers." An added problem is the fact many of these restaurant owners don't even know for sure where their fish is coming from, so they cannot tell their customers what they are actually eating.

Solving the food fraud problem will require efforts at local, federal, and even international levels who are charged with monitoring the supply chain, spotting fraud when it happens either unintentionally or intentionally (i.e., identifying criminal networks profiting from food fraud), correcting the problem, and vigorously holding any true fraudsters accountable. For the average consumer, however, the best defense against this fraud is to stick with reputable suppliers of food from the choices in the market to the restaurants you patronize. Know where your food is coming from. Ask questions. And when in doubt, take it out of your diet.

The cruel irony about food-related conditions is that we live in increasingly high-tech times with access to revolutionary medical therapies and opportunities to eat whatever we want whenever we want. In Western society, we don't worry so much about potable water supplies, famine, and communicable diseases. But considerable questions swirl around the allergy/ intolerance debate: Why do some people seem to inherit problems with certain foods, whereas others develop them without a family history? Does where you were born and where you live today factor into the equation? You bet.

DOES GEOGRAPHIC LOCATION MATTER?

One of the more perplexing characteristics about food allergies is the disparate rate across populations in the world. The prevalence and patterns of food allergy appear highly variable in different parts of the world, although it's important to note that high-quality studies have not been conducted in many regions and much of the data overall are focused on pediatric allergy. We are just getting started in our endeavors as epidemiologists to chronicle the world's allergy epidemic across all nations and ages.

Our global estimates are based on limited research samples, which may not paint a complete picture though future research will help us fill in the blanks. Although most food allergy research to date has primarily been conducted in Australia, North America, and Europe, we're beginning to collect data from Asia, Africa, the Middle East, and Central and South America to help paint a more comprehensive picture and provide that 30,000-foot view of evidence. Understanding why certain countries have much higher rates of food allergies than others will help clue us into the reasons for the epidemic and how to solve it.

What we know so far is that estimated rates are higher in the US, Australia, and the UK than in Greece and Spain, but the reason remains a mystery and we don't think it's attributed to different diets. What's really interesting is that studies on childhood food allergy in particular found baffling disparities: the overall prevalence of food allergy in kids under five years of age was only 1 percent in Thailand, but as high as 5.3 percent in Korean infants and 10 percent in Australian preschoolers. Again, we're not sure why. Also, the questions asked and methods for collecting these data were not the same in all countries.

Adding to this conundrum is noting that the allergen culprits themselves can vary widely. Interestingly, the most common food allergens in a specific country are often the most common foods eaten there. For example, hazelnut is common in France, whereas chickpea is common in India. In Israel, sesame seed is one of the most common allergens as well as a leading cause of anaphylaxis. Furthermore, the prevalence of allergies can vary widely among countries within the same continent. For example, milk and egg are the most common allergens in early childhood in the UK, US, Australia, and many parts of Europe and Asia. Case in point: the so-called EuroPrevall birth study, which recruited more than twelve thousand infants from nine European centers with different climatic and cultural backgrounds, found that the incidence of cow's milk allergy was lower in southeastern European countries, such as Greece and Italy, compared to the UK and Netherlands. The pervasiveness of egg allergy was also highly variable—the lowest incidence was again reported in more southern countries.

Moving around the world, we find that the most common food allergens in Asia are also different from those seen in Western countries. Peanut allergy predominates in children under five years of age in the UK, US, and Australia, but is very uncommon in the rest of Asia apart from Japan. In a geographic study of the US, we found peanut allergy to be higher in urban areas compared to rural areas. The only specific food allergy that was equally common across population density in the US was milk allergy.

In Thailand, Japan, and Korea, wheat is becoming one of the most common food allergens in childhood, followed by egg and milk. A large study in Korea found that walnuts were the most common cause of food allergy in preschoolers and school-age children, whereas buckwheat and wheat allergy were most common in adolescents. And just as shellfish has been documented to be a leading cause of food allergy in adolescents and adults in the US, it's also increasingly documented in other parts of Asia. What explains all these staggering imbalances?

One of the first areas of interest for research scientists like me in pursuit of solving this giant puzzle has been looking at migration patterns. And, lo and behold, we've discovered that Australian-born children with an Asian parent have higher rates of nut allergy than do kids born in Asia who migrate to Australia. Such a finding suggests the Asian environment is somehow protective against food allergy, but Asian children born in Australia are at much higher risk of developing food allergies. Why? Possible reasons could be because those Australian-born Asian children have been exposed to a different environment. And by "environment," I'm not only referring to the climate and UV sunlight exposure, but also diet and even microbial exposures that factor mightily into the microbiome.

Timing of migration also could be having an impact. When parents move out of Asia *after the early infant period*, their children appear to be at less risk of developing food allergies, especially nut allergy. This pattern has been shown to be the case in North America as well. Put simply, when families migrate across countries and continents with young kids, typically under the age of five, those children face a higher risk for developing allergic diseases than do their peers whose families moved when they were older. The highest risk is among infants born in the new Westernized country. They hold the highest risk, which may be due to the fact they did not get the exposure to the protective environment or food in early life.

My colleagues at the Murdoch Children's Research Institute in Melbourne, who documented the Asia-Australia data, and which encompassed more than fifty-seven thousand five-year-olds, also revealed that children from urban areas are more likely to have nut allergy than do kids from rural regions. This is similar to what we have documented here in the US. A 2013 study I described previously in *JAMA Pediatrics* found that foreign-born children who live in the US have a lower risk of developing allergies—but, even more interesting, their risk for allergies *increases* the longer they remain here. Kids of immigrants born in the US develop food allergies at a much higher rate. This is my personal story and a story I hear repeatedly. What is lost in the environment of Asian-born children early in life that causes them to be even more susceptible to developing allergies? If we can pinpoint these missing pieces, we could potentially help all children prevent allergies. Again, the million-dollar question! If you have ideas, please feel free to write and share. It takes all of us investigating to truly find answers.

I've painted a confusing picture, I know, but welcome to my (exciting) world. This is a giant puzzle my colleagues and I are trying to figure out. We in the scientific world have only begun to scratch the surface of the science behind food allergies, and our understanding of the populations who are at highest risk of becoming food allergic. As my colleagues and I continue to piece together global data, we are finding that allergies are more interconnected than we think.

Generally speaking, while we all know that our environment—our lifestyle choices, such as what we eat and how we exercise—plays a significant role in our health, we often don't think about the subtler forms of "environment" that have an impact on us, such as our geographical location and whether we've moved from a different country or even a different state. It's likely that differences in food allergy patterns around the world are attributed to a complex interplay of genetic, epigenetic, and environmental factors. There is also remarkable variability in food allergy risk among different ethnic groups within the same country. In South Africa, for instance, black African (Xhosa) children have a significantly lower prevalence of peanut allergy compared to children of mixed race origin (Caucasian and Black). African American and Latinx children living in the US, however, have significantly higher odds of food allergy, asthma, and eczema compared to white children. How do we explain these discrepancies?

Again, it's a complex interplay of forces, from early life exposures and feeding patterns in infants to genetic vulnerabilities and racial disparities in health care. We are just beginning to understand how race and ethnicity play an important role in how people are affected by food allergy. It wasn't until 2016 that the first study documenting different food allergy profiles across African American, white, and Latinx children and teens was published in the *Journal of Allergy and Clinical Immunology*. The researchers, myself included with others at Rush University and Cincinnati Children's Hospital, found that African American kids have significantly higher odds of allergy to wheat, soy, corn, fish, and shellfish compared to their white (non-Latinx) peers; and Latinx children have significantly higher odds of allergy to corn, fish, and shellfish, but a similar rate of asthma compared to non-Latinx white children. Peanut was the most common food allergen in all three groups. The only allergen more common among white children than African American and Latinx children was tree nut. My colleagues and I pointed out that the elevated rate of corn allergy observed in the Latinx community could be due to corn being a major food staple in their culture.

But the overall discovery of these disproportionate allergy rates among African American and Latinx children compared to white kids, coupled with higher odds of emergency room visits and food-induced anaphylaxis in these communities (compared to white children), is cause for concern. The previously dominant narrative that food allergy is more common in middle to high income white populations is simply not true. Not only are other races and ethnicities affected, but they could be uniquely vulnerable and suffering even more due to fewer resources, less access to education around food allergy, and deep divides in health-care access. This is true for both children and adults. It goes without saying that in our study, we concluded that we need to develop culturally sensitive and effective educational programs to improve food allergy outcomes for all.

There's much more to this geographic story. Ecological studies have identified several climatic factors, such as latitude, sunlight exposure, and season of birth, correlating with vitamin D status, as well as ambient humidity, as potential geographic determinants that may control food allergy risk in infancy. This is true on an international as well as more microcosmic scale. In the US, for example, there's variability by states, possibly due to differences in diet, vitamin D levels, what pollens are in the air, or even whether one is living near the coast or not. And just when you thought this picture could not get any more convoluted, believe it or not, culinary practices could also be having an impact and changing risk profiles throughout the world. Roasted peanuts, which are common in a Western diet, are more likely to trigger allergies compared to peanuts that are boiled or fried, which is practiced more often in Asian cuisine. Treating peanuts with food additives, such as vinegar in Korea, has also been shown to reduce risk of peanut allergies. Moreover, let's not forget that some places, such as France, have the highest allergies to foods most common in their diet, such as hazelnuts. Other studies show foods prominent in the diet from an early age may prevent allergies. The complexity on the spectrum of adverse food reactions grows deeper.

The fact environmental forces as diverse as diet and geography (how close you live to the equator, for instance) can influence risk for allergies cannot be understated. I defined epigenetics in a previous chapter (changes in gene expression without changes to the underlying DNA sequence), but it bears reiterating that how any physical body behaves—all the way down to its molecular structure—is heavily influenced by epigenetic drivers. Epigenetic forces help explain why identical twins can grow up to look and behave somewhat differently from each other and why each possesses a different assortment of risk factors, despite harboring precisely the same DNA sequence. Their DNA may be identical, but the sum of epigenetic changes that they acquire in response to their environment throughout life alters how their identical DNA is expressed.

When it comes to solving problems in medicine, I'm an eternal optimist. As you can tell from this first part of the book, my colleagues and I have a lot of work to do but I'm excited by the task at hand and feel honored to be in the position I find myself in daily to help families and individuals gain freedom from their fear of food while I also hunt down more clues to the epidemic. It's an intricate tapestry for sure, but the beauty of it is that I get to toggle between the hard-core data in my epidemiological lab work and engaging with real people who bring colorful experiences from their lives to my talks and clinical practice. I reap all of my inspiration from families and their stories and passion. They never give up, and neither will I. Working with families is my "little incubator of ideas," which gives me the opportunity to understand first-hand where the big holes in research are. And then I can leap toward those holes and aim to fill them.

Hopefully, Part 1 gave you a sweeping view of the spectrum, especially with regard to addressing the drivers of the food allergy epidemic and all its nuances, masqueraders included. For most people dealing with allergic diseases, the first question is not why, but *what*—what kind of food-related conditions do they have? Is it a real allergy or masquerader? How can they find out for sure what their symptoms mean and what they can do about it? Turn the page and enter Part 2 where I cover everything you need to know about diagnosing and treating any food-related condition on the spectrum and learning how to live life fully. You, too, can be part of the cure not just for yourself but for the world.

Fearless Facts

➔ Modern labeling practices in the food industry need more attention and clarification.

➔ Claims on the front, such as "vegan," "dairy-free," etc., are not covered by the Food Allergen Labeling and Consumer Protection Act (FALCPA); always read the ingredients and "contains . . ." box (if this is available).

➔ The FALCPA requires that food labels clearly identify the food source names of any ingredients that are "major food allergens" or contain any protein derived from a "major food allergen," which includes the following nine common allergens: milk, eggs, fish (e.g., bass, flounder, cod), crustacean shellfish (e.g., crab, lobster, shrimp), tree nuts (e.g., almonds, walnuts, pecans), peanuts, wheat, soybeans, and sesame. Note that molluscan shellfish—such as oysters, clams, mussels, or scallops—are not required to be labeled as a major allergens.

➔ The FALCPA's labeling requirements do not apply to the potential or unintentional presence of major food allergens in foods resulting from "cross-contact" situations during manufacturing.

➔ Companies may use precautionary allergen labeling (PAL) on packaging to label products for which there is a risk of cross-contact with food allergens during production. But, unfortunately, such measures remain *voluntary* and *unregulated*, and such labeling is inconsistent.

➔ Organic and GMO foods are not inherently allergen-free.

✢ Processed foods can hide food allergens that escape clear labeling, or their ingredients are disguised by other terms used to refer to, say, milk proteins or egg.

✢ Food additives and naturally occurring chemicals in many foods ("food agents") can also be problematic and contribute to conditions across the spectrum.

✢ Geography matters: Where you live in the world, your ethnic origin, and migration timing from birth to adulthood each play a role in determining your risk of developing conditions across the spectrum of food reactions.

PART II

FINDING FOOD FREEDOM

Identify and Empower; Treat;

Manage and Prevent; and Thrive

six

IDENTIFY AND EMPOWER

How to Make Sense of Imperfect Testing Methods

Hippocrates, the father of Western medicine, once quipped, "It is far more important to know what person the disease has than what disease the person has." He is often credited with first recognizing that food could be responsible for adverse symptoms and even death in some individuals. In his writings (460–377 BC), he referred to the presence of "hostile humors" (possibly IgE antibodies) in some men that made them "suffer badly" following ingestion of cheese. If only Hippocrates could see the food allergy world today (or any area of medicine, really). Our field of food allergy research has made exponential strides over the past two millennia. But despite our many advances, plenty of gaps in our knowledge still keep scientists, like me, up at night.

Testing for diabetes is well defined. Checking someone's temperature can be done in seconds, without even touching the individual. And confirming a pregnancy only takes a couple of minutes. But diagnosing food allergies and their masquerading counterparts? This process is anything but simple, reliable, quick, or efficient. Compared with other conditions, food-related problems is an area of medicine still in its infancy as their incidences have increased so much over the past twenty years. Research is moving fast and new diagnostics are currently being developed and tested. That's why the cornerstone of our management plan is Identify. And once you identify the source of your food-related issues, you can then Empower yourself with the knowledge to move forward and find the right treatment and management protocol. I may have painted a not-too-rosy, imperfect perspective of diagnostics on the food allergy spectrum, but there's hope in new science and plenty of current tactics to help anyone through the maze.

In this chapter, I'm going to explore the main methods of testing so you're prepared for working with a professional and are Empowered to Manage and Treat your condition (and Prevent new allergies, as much as possible). You may have already been diagnosed and merely seek additional information and further confirmation that you're on the right track with your or your loved one's food issues. Or perhaps you're questioning the accuracy of a diagnosis and want more assurance because you have doubts, or you've been told to avoid a whole category of foods you love. Often, after getting tested for a number of foods, people refrain from eating certain items when in fact they were never allergic to them to begin with. Importantly, blood tests and skin prick tests are most useful with a detailed history like the one you filled out in the beginning of this book. You will also learn more about the STOP method in this chapter, to help prepare you if you ever experience a reaction. Testing alone without the history can even open the door to what's called the "nocebo effect" whereby you *think* you have an adverse reaction to a particular food and have a psychosomatic response to it, but there's no underlying medical cause. Studies show that some people who avoid gluten, for example, because they think their digestive issues are a result of that ingredient when they have no real health reason to do so, could be under the spell of the nocebo effect. All the press around gluten that has tainted its image is enough to set off a very real negative physical response in some people after they've consumed it. Nocebo ("I will harm") is the placebo ("I will please") effect's evil twin.

Another matter complicating this picture is the fact that there are so many possible diagnoses—from IgE-mediated reactions to non-IgE-mediated reactions—many of which share common symptoms and food triggers. Unlike, say, being pregnant, which rarely has a gray area (i.e., you're either pregnant or you're not), the food allergy world is one giant gray field open to interpretation, lack of definitive testing, and changes over time as a person's biology shifts with age, history, and new exposures. We also cannot neglect adverse reactions that are not classified as food allergy but do indeed take up space on the spectrum. Those masqueraders, for example, can be difficult to tease out and complicate the diagnostic endeavor. But again, this is when science can lead the way. No matter where you are in your journey, this chapter will help you to understand the science behind identifying various problems on the spectrum and knowing what to do next that makes sense for you and your condition.

I'll start by saying that there are many nuances to testing that require the attention of a qualified doctor who will work with you and give you the knowledge—and facts—you need to make the best decisions for yourselves and your loved ones. This is one of those areas in medicine where there is not a one-size-fits-all solution. Each patient must be considered within the context of his or her age, lifestyle, environment, and family dynamics. And the first step in this process is distinguishing between immunologic (immune-based) and nonimmunologic (non-immune-based) reactions. Let's get to it.

FOOD ALLERGY TESTING IS A COLLABORATIVE EFFORT

Currently, no single universal method adequately meets the usual safety, sensitivity, and specificity required to diagnose a food allergy. The diagnosis of food allergy is primarily based on a combination of a patient's medical history, skin prick/scratch tests where appropriate, certain lab work to identify the presence of IgE antibodies, elimination diets (removing certain foods from one's diet and then possibly reintroducing them later and noting any changes/effects), and oral food challenges. The food challenges still remain the gold standard for diagnosing an IgE-mediated food allergy, but it can be time-intensive and scary for some due to the risk of a severe reaction. Costs and access can be a major issue too.

What's so important about diagnosing food allergies and related conditions correctly is that management differs, and it is important to know whether the condition is treatable and whether it is potentially severe. There's no reason to refrain from foods—and their nutrients—if you're not allergic or sensitive to them. This is why it behooves people to work with a board-certified allergist who is specifically trained to administer and to interpret food allergy tests. The spectrum of adverse food reactions, as you've learned by now, is both wide and deep.

Remember, a reaction to a certain ingredient may not qualify as a food allergy because it does not incite the immune system, but it's nonetheless troublesome and reduces one's quality of life. What's more, adverse food reactions can manifest—and masquerade—in a number of chronic conditions that share similar and overlapping symptoms. If you think, for example, that microwave and movie-theater popcorn triggers migraines, wouldn't it be nice to know that it's not the popcorn itself but the dye (tartrazine) used to make the snack yellow? You'd be able to make better choices in the popcorn department and not nix the food entirely from your life. Misdiagnosing a food allergy or intolerance can cause a person to unnecessarily evict many foods from their diet and miss out on diet balance and diversity—both of which are key to health. Put another way, if you aren't properly diagnosed, you could be skipping foods that you need for adequate nutrition (and that you'd enjoy!).

Does the following sound familiar? You have a bad reaction to one food and are anxious to know what other foods you should avoid. So, you purchase over-the-counter sensitivity kits and the results come back with a laundry list of potentially "bad" foods due to the presence of antibodies to those foods. And then you subsequently avoid them even though you were never diagnosed as allergic to many of them. Thankfully, new blood tests are in development that hope to be more accurate in their nature for identifying which molecules within foods are causing the problems. This will help people avoid nixing entire swathes of nutritious foods when they only need to avoid a small number of them.

Do Not DIY

One important message I want to state clearly is that self-diagnosing should be avoided. I know it can be tempting, especially with the explosion of at-home lab testing kits sold in your local drugstore or online (at the time of writing, do-it-yourself testing kits cost anywhere from about $35 for an individual test to $450 for a battery of tests; it's a multi-billion-dollar market that you've certainly been exposed to through media at some point). These kits are not FDA-regulated, and while they can seem like an initial source of empowering information without the hassle of going to a doctor, suspected food allergies should always be evaluated, diagnosed, and treated by a qualified medical professional. Many kits rely on looking at IgG levels (as opposed to IgE levels; I'll get into this more in a bit), but those IgG levels can be elevated without indicating an allergy—which results in a lot of false positives. There's nothing empowering about receiving the wrong diagnosis. And these kits won't help if you are dealing with some of the masqueraders or are on the farther right of the spectrum where other conditions complicate the picture. If you don't Identify right, you cannot Treat or Manage correctly and find freedom.

The other big concern about these kits is how to act on the information they reveal. Without training in allergy, someone might not use the information correctly. Translating test results into meaningful recommendations to patients is hard enough for doctors. Complicating diagnoses further is the fact that food allergies are a moving target as we age and our physiology changes. Many children with allergies to milk, eggs, wheat, dairy, and soy outgrow them, usually by about age five. But only about 10 to 20 percent of those with allergies to peanuts, tree nuts, and shellfish do. And for reasons not fully understood, patients—especially adults—can develop allergies they've previously tolerated, particularly shellfish.

False Positives in the Doctor's Office

During the week I was working on this very chapter, I went to my primary care provider for a yearly checkup. We discussed my work and she confirmed that at least 1 in 5, if not more, of her patients said they were avoiding a food and thought they may have a food allergy or food condition. Interestingly, we proceeded to discuss testing and the best ways to diagnose.

Allergy testing is not foolproof even in doctors' offices. Because of the high rates of false positives with current blood tests, without a good clear history, these tests can be confusing even to the general clinician. We have highly predictive lab values to only a handful of allergens. It does someone little good to find out that they're sensitized to peanuts, pets, or pollen if it doesn't cause a medical problem. But it could cause people to drastically change their diet and lifestyle to the point they lose out on comprehensive nutrition, or needlessly lose a beloved dog, or avoid the outdoors. For a long time, a panel test that tested for a number of common allergens was being promoted for primary care. Now, there is a big push to stop random panels and focus on history as the driving force for testing specific foods individually. This is also why it's important to work with your primary care doctors and an allergist so that proper diagnoses can be made and, if multiple food allergies are diagnosed, any nutritional deficits from avoiding so many foods can also be addressed. If you are not diagnosed with a true allergy and sit somewhere on the spectrum where you're having mixed reactions or another potential food-related condition that does not involve the immune system, a proper diagnosis will enable you to find the correct practitioner.

Studies in recent years have shown that a huge portion of blood and skin prick tests that come back positive for peanut allergy among children, for example, may not in fact indicate a true peanut allergy (this is what we refer to as a false positive): kids in these studies were found not to be allergic upon a food challenge and could eat peanuts without a reaction. In 2020, researchers from the University of Manchester performed food challenges with seventy-nine children who had positive skin or blood tests for peanut allergy. An astounding 66 percent of them were found not to be allergic. The findings, published in the *Journal of Allergy and Clinical Immunology*, confirmed two studies released in 2007 out of Sydney Children's and Johns Hopkins Hospitals reporting large discrepancies in the results of skin and blood tests for peanut allergies. Our own studies corroborate these findings. False positives are not just a problem in pediatric allergy testing—adults can be equally deceived by unreliable test results, leading to unnecessary and potentially harmful dietary changes. When it's stated about 50 percent of all blood tests and skin prick tests will yield a "false positive" result, that figure relates with people of all ages. The test alone cannot be thought of as conclusive without a strong positive history of a reaction to the food, in this case peanut. The good news is that recent studies have found that new blood tests, including peanut components and epitope mapping, may provide a much more reliable diagnostic to certain food allergies, such as peanut. Also, a food allergy can be confirmed with a food challenge, which we will discuss.

Without a clear understanding of what exactly a person is allergic to—or not—it's hard to know what to do and how to navigate foods. It's a case where a little knowledge can do more harm than good.

MEDICAL HISTORY—THE MOST IMPORTANT FIRST STEP

When you visit an allergist for a diagnosis, you will walk through several steps (you may have done this already at some point). The first one is simple: despite all the fancy technology we have now at our disposal, nothing beats an old-school medical history during which the patient explains their experiences with food. For some, they know exactly what's troubling them because they can link a reaction to the consumption of an obvious culprit. If you break out into hives every time you eat anything with peanuts in it, you can probably surmise that peanut is the causative food. Other allergies can be more challenging to pinpoint. Remember, too, that food—whether whole, fresh, or processed—is a complex entity. Not only are we dealing with multiple ingredients (and molecules) within any given product, but there's always the possibility of cross-contact and cross-reactivity.

Keeping notes or a food journal/diary on your allergy experience is key for when you'll need to answer important questions, such as:

→ Which food(s) give you trouble? What ingredients or items are suspect?
→ Were you able to eat the food before? In a different form? If so, how much, how often, and when was the last time (days, weeks, or months ago)?
→ How were the food(s) prepared (e.g., raw, baked, cooked, marinated)?
→ How would you describe your symptoms?
→ Are any medications taken around the same time?
→ How long after you eat the food(s) do the symptoms show up and resolve?
→ How much of the food(s) did you eat?
→ How often do you get the reaction? Every time you eat the food(s)? Are there other circumstances that seem to be related, such as having a reaction at a meal after exercise or during a menstrual cycle?
→ What type of treatments have you had, if any (whether self-treated or professionally)?

I've included a sample blank food log in Appendix C. The more information you can provide, the better for guiding future tests. Even photos—selfies—of a reaction can help. A complete exam should also include questions about diet, family medical history, and the home environment. If there's a lot of ragweed pollen in the air, for example, and you have an oral allergy syndrome whereby you experience swelling or itching in your mouth and throat if you eat certain foods, such as melon, these circumstances need to all be factored into the diagnosis. This type of food-related condition on the spectrum—pollen-food allergy syndrome (PFAS)—which I defined earlier, is often misdiagnosed as an extreme food allergy and thus is a masquerader. PFAS is an immune-based reaction and so it's technically an allergy, but it rarely leads to anaphylaxis.

Once a comprehensive medical history has been established, the next step is testing when warranted by the history.

Second opinions: Not all allergists are created equal. If you doubt a diagnosis or feel that your doctor is not listening to you and your experience, seek a second opinion. More on this on page 162.

SKIN PRICK TESTS (SPTs)

A skin prick or skin scratch test (SPT) is just what it sounds like: it entails scratching a person's skin (usually on the forearms or back) with a tiny bit of liquid extract of an allergen, such as pollen or food. Sometimes fresh food, such as fruits, vegetables, and seafood may be used instead of a solution. There are many different scratch test devices an allergist may use, based on preferences and other factors. Often employing a metal or plastic device, they provide an "epicutaneous" scratch of the skin surface to introduce a small concentration of the allergen. Following a waiting period of usually fifteen to twenty minutes or so, the doctor will note the formation of redness and raised, clear swelling areas (called wheals, similar to what a mosquito bite looks like), measure them, and use these data to inform their food allergy diagnosis. An SPT is typically interpreted as positive if the wheal diameter is 3 mm greater than a saline negative control. Of note, intradermal testing of food allergens, injected below the skin with a needle, has no role in diagnosing and treating food allergy. In fact, intradermal testing may induce multiple false positive reactions and can provoke serious allergic reactions in some instances.

The advantages of SPTs are that they are simple, inexpensive, noninvasive, and the results can be obtained quickly. The shortcoming is that there can be false positives without a good, detailed medical history in hand. Sometimes, members of a food "family" often share similar proteins. For example, if you are allergic to peanuts, your tests may show a positive response to other members of the legume family, such as green peas, even if eating green peas has never been a problem for you. This is called cross-reactivity. The test is positive because it recognizes a similar protein in peanuts and green peas. But the test hasn't detected the real culprit—a different, unique protein that is found only in peanuts.

False negatives can also occur for multiple reasons, though they are uncommon. One reason is that the act of scratching did not introduce enough allergen to trigger a skin response. In general, the larger the reaction, the more likely that the diagnosis of food allergy is clinically relevant; but larger values do not correlate with severity of reactions (in other words, size is not an accurate predictor of how severe an allergic reaction might be). And multiple variables can affect the outcome, from the nature of the allergen (commercial extracts or fresh foods) to the technique the health-care professional uses (e.g., pressure, body location, timing of measurement, sensitive skin). Because the test depends on the release of histamine from sensitized mast cells, it may be suppressed or blocked for those who take antihistamines and cannot discontinue them before testing. Other medications can also potentially interfere with test results, such as oral steroids, Singulair, and antacids. So, while SPTs have inherent limitations, they have value when used by an experienced allergist in the context of the medical history and they provide a gateway for further testing.

BLOOD TESTS

These tests measure the presence of IgE antibodies to specific foods (again, IgE is short for "immunoglobulin E"; it is the antibody that triggers food allergy symptoms). Not all food allergies that occur involve IgE, as I've described. IgE can be classified as specific for certain foods or environmental triggers. This is called specific IgE (sIgE) and is measured on a scale of 0 to >100 kUA/L (kilo units of allergen per liter). Wide ranges are noted and various levels that may or may not correlate with food allergy.

In general, the higher the IgE values to a specific food, the more likely it represents a risk of IgE-mediated food allergy. But this is not always the case and detailed medical/food history needs to accompany the IgE. Also, the level of sIgE does not predict clinical severity. Some people may have extremely high sIgE levels yet have minor reactions, and others with low sIgE levels have severe reactions with exposed foods. Also, some food-specific IgE measurements are more likely to cause symptoms at lower values compared to others.

To further complicate the matter, even in patients who can tolerate foods, sometimes specific IgE values may be measurable. This would be considered a false positive and doesn't necessarily mean that you have to remove the foods from your diet. Levels of specific IgE along with a good, detailed history can help your physician determine the next steps in diagnosing food allergy.

In non-IgE food allergy, one's allergic symptoms may be triggered by factors that can't be measured, and the blood test that comes back "negative" for an IgE measurement. An IgE-mediated milk allergy will typically be revealed by a positive blood test, but a non-IgE-mediated allergy or lactose intolerance will not be represented by the blood test result.

Specific IgE can be broken down into "component" testing. Remember that specific IgE is measuring certain proteins that are circulating in your blood, some of which have no clinical relevance for symptoms. With component IgE testing, the identification of clinically relevant allergens in the foods can be identified and measured; that is, the specific part(s) of the allergen that prompt a reaction. This type of testing is called component resolved diagnosis (CRD). Component testing is available for milk, egg, wheat, soy, peanut, cashew, hazelnut, walnut, Brazil nut, red meat (alpha-gal), and in some research centers allergens associated with PFAS can be measured. The importance of CRD testing is that it can determine some specific allergies with improved accuracy and also help rule out false positives on IgE measurements.

Suffice it to say these immunoglobulin tests are not foolproof, which is why I stress the importance of working with a medical professional well versed in this area to help you decide which tests are best and how to interpret their results. Knowing and respecting the limitations of these tests is part of Empowering yourself. In many areas of medicine, in fact, tests are *clues*—not answers. And in the food allergy space, immunoglobin testing can provide unclear clues. It's important to underscore that panels of blood tests are not recommended by allergists due to all these complications that don't paint a clear and definitive picture and could be misleading. I repeat: If you test positive to a food you are eating in your diet, you are not allergic to it though you are sensitized to it. You should keep it in your diet and not begin avoiding it. As you know now, there are exceptions to every rule and here it is: EoE, which we will also discuss (see page 150).

As I called out previously, ordering "food sensitivity tests" online is not advised. Many of these websites selling DIY test kits report using IgG tests, for example, to look for another type of antibody and determine which foods you should avoid (and suggest help with symptoms beyond just allergies, from IBS and obesity to autism); these tests are very confusing and do not always do what they claim to do. Immunoglobulin G (IgG) is another class of immunoglobulin that is the most common antibody found in blood circulation—composing about 75 percent of blood antibodies in humans. It's also found in extracellular fluid. IgG's main job is to bind to many kinds of pathogens, such as viruses, bacteria, and fungi, to protect the body from infection. These antibodies may be involved in reactions to food proteins that they "see" as potentially harmful like a pathogen. What this means is that IgG levels can elevate simply because you eat a specific food, so it doesn't necessarily mean that your body is reacting negatively (hence a lot of false positives).

There are many different types of blood tests on the market and different laboratories sometimes use different "brands" of tests, each of which report using slightly different scoring systems or units. For this reason, I reiterate that it's important to work with your primary care physician and an experienced allergist who is familiar with these tests and their variability. Although blood and skin prick tests offer information about the chance of a food allergy, they cannot predict the severity of an allergy. New diagnostics are being developed with the hopes of a more accurate diagnosis and determination of severity.

ELIMINATION DIETS

The elimination diet generally lasts two to four weeks. During this period, a patient avoids the suspect foods and records and reports symptoms to their doctor. If one or more of these foods is causing a reaction of some sort, symptoms should disappear by the end of this period. In some cases, the doctor may add another step, gradually reintroducing a problem food to the diet. If symptoms return, it is likely that the food (or something in that food such as an additive) is causing the response. This method, combined with skin or blood tests, can be helpful in diagnosing both IgE-mediated food allergies and masqueraders, such as intolerances that affect the gut (e.g., nonceliac gluten sensitivity, lactose intolerance).

It cannot be understated: Food is complicated, making diagnosing food-related conditions all the more complicated!

ORAL FOOD CHALLENGES (OFCs)

Dr. S. Allan Bock is fondly known as one of the pioneers of oral food challenges; he also happens to be a dear colleague and mentor of mine who has since retired after spending decades at National Jewish Health in Denver, Colorado—a leading hospital and research center. I will never forget how Dr. Bock was one of the first to believe in me when I was starting my career and presenting at the national conference. He took me under his wing and we would meet for mentoring sessions every year; he continues to be a source of wisdom. Working with nationally renowned pediatrician Charles D. May in the 1970s, who Dr. Bock calls the father of scientific food allergy, Bock helped perfect the procedure of the double-blind, placebo-controlled food challenge and made it the gold standard for the evaluation of adverse reactions to foods. "I was lucky to be in the right place at the right time," Bock says. He has written extensively on food hypersensitivity; his book *Food Allergy: A Primer for People* was published in 1988 and was among the first to cover the topic.

At the start of his career forty-five years ago, food allergy was a backwater of medical research. The condition was rare and poorly understood. Under Charles May's tutelage, Dr. Bock and another young investigator then at Duke University, Dr. Hugh Sampson, helped define the biological nature of food allergies and finally ground the food allergy field in science-based medicine. In a food challenge, patients are fed tiny, then increasing, amounts of food and closely monitored for any allergic reactions. This helped sort out what was truly an allergic reaction to food and what was often caused by other things such as medications, allergen exposures by inhalation or contact, viral illness, exercise, or even panic. I'm honored to also count Dr. Sampson among my colleagues today; he is the Kurt Hirschhorn Professor of Pediatrics at the Icahn School of Medicine at Mount Sinai and Director Emeritus of the Jaffe Food Allergy Institute.

A pediatric allergist, immunologist, and father of three daughters (one of whom had an egg allergy), Dr. Sampson has been helping patients manage their food allergies for decades and continues to search for better diagnostics and treatments. He is optimistic about the future of food allergy: "We've seen food allergy turned into a science. There's tremendous interest in understanding basic biology and diagnostics, and now that many bright and talented people are entering and working in this field like never before, new things will come along." As someone who once had to "talk about food allergy in the restroom at conferences" because medicine hadn't yet recognized it as a bona fide condition worthy of investigation, he's as excited about the future of food allergy medicine as I am.

I also agree with him that "Over time treatment will get better incrementally—think evolution, not revolution." Until better diagnostics emerge, the oral food challenge remains an important tool. Because this test can cause a serious allergic reaction, only an experienced allergist should conduct it. It can be time-consuming, expensive, and nerve-racking, especially for people who have witnessed someone encounter a life-threatening reaction in which breathing becomes difficult or, worse, multiple organs begin to shut down. Hence, it should happen at a medical facility with the appropriate medications and equipment at the ready.

During the food challenge, the allergist feeds the patient the suspect food in measured doses. He or she will start with very small amounts that are unlikely to trigger symptoms. With each dose, the health-care professional will watch the patient for a period of time for any signs of a reaction. If there are no significant symptoms, the patient will gradually receive larger and larger doses. If signs of a reaction surface, however, the food challenge will stop. With OFCs, most reactions are mild, such as flushing or hives, but severe reactions can happen and therefore the physician is ready, observing closely with epinephrine at hand. Because of the potential for a serious reaction, the benefit of a challenge has to be carefully weighed against the risk. Some people are fine undergoing this type of test, but for others, the thought of eating something (say, an egg) that's been avoided for more than a decade, the prospect of facing a serious reaction is too unappealing. It's easier to just continue to avoid the food.

There are different types of oral food challenges. The open OFC involves ingestion of the food in a commonly encountered form (such as peanut butter), with both the patient and the doctor aware of the challenge food. In a single-blinded OFC, the food is administered in a masked form (either in a capsule or mixed with another food to hide the flavor and texture) and the doctor (but not the patient) is aware of the food being challenged. On the other hand, the double-blind, placebo-controlled food challenge, which is the gold standard for a definite confirmation of food allergy, involves administration of the food so that neither the doctor nor the patient knows whether the food they are being challenged with is a placebo or an allergen. In OFCs, the food must first be completely eliminated from the diet for at least two weeks prior to the challenge.

Although oral food challenges can be scary, they also can lead to next steps in terms of arriving at a definitive diagnosis and then treatment. I'll never forget the oral food challenge my daughter underwent to egg when she was three years old. We were asked to bring the food we were introducing, so I made a cheese omelet and took it to the appointment. I learned how hard this can be on the other side when you are a loved one watching carefully for a reaction after every bite. How exciting it feels when there is no reaction as they consume increasing amounts of the food; then, leaving and going home thrilled your beloved has passed the challenge and can add another food item to their diet. Or, in the scenario where the food challenge pinpoints the presence of a serious food allergy, novel treatments, such as oral immunotherapy, can be considered to train the immune system to tolerate slowly increasing amounts.

Studies show that regardless of whether an individual passes or fails a food challenge, the result nevertheless improves quality of life because it provides key information: you actually know whether you are really allergic or not. That old adage rings true: information is power. It informs not only where you stand, but what you can do next. Also, if you do have a reaction and need to receive epinephrine, it makes you more comfortable with future use of epinephrine and again improves your quality of life. If in doubt about whether you truly have a food allergy, it is wise to discuss a food challenge with your allergist.

In the future, we may not have to resort to oral food challenges at all as we develop better testing, including predictive biomarker tests, components, and epitope mapping for detecting allergies and their severity. Imagine a simple blood test that can tell you exactly what your allergens are with almost 100 percent accuracy. These revolutionary diagnostics are in experimental phases, but are showing promising results that will change the food allergy landscape in our lifetime for everyone—infants to older adults. Other tests that can look at certain genes involved in an allergic response will also play a role. We may not be able to change an actual gene in a person that impacts risk for allergy, but perhaps we can change how the gene *functions*—truly twenty-first-century medicine. This is the essence of epigenetic medicine, or being able to influence how our static DNA behaves in its dynamic expression in the body. And it's also the heart of precision medicine, which personalizes an individual's unique treatment to his or her own physiology. We can finally turn diagnostics from a dilemma to a definitive protocol.

MASKED MASQUERADERS: MIXED FOOD ALLERGY

Mixed food allergy disorders are characterized by both IgE-dependent and IgE-independent mechanisms that affect the skin (atopic dermatitis) and gastrointestinal tract (eosinophilic gastrointestinal disorders, known as EGIDs). Eosinophilic esophagitis (EoE), and EGIDs, including eosinophilic gastritis (EG), eosinophilic gastroenteritis (EGE), and eosinophilic colitis (EC), are characterized by chronic inflammation of the esophagus, stomach, small intestine, and colon, respectively, with increases in the numbers of eosinophils on biopsy. People with these disorders can experience a spectrum of symptoms, from generalized abdominal pain to difficulty swallowing food, impaction of food, vomiting, and diarrhea. And because they can have many overlapping symptoms with other (unrelated) conditions, I call them the masked masqueraders.

Patients with EGIDs often do have other allergies, such as atopic dermatitis and asthma, but other conditions that can result in the same symptoms must be ruled out, including parasitic infections, inflammatory bowel disease (IBD), and some cancers. Above all else, working with an experienced GI doctor is imperative to identify these conditions. For patients with multiple allergic issues (asthma, rhinitis, food allergy, eczema) and chronic GI symptoms lasting more than three weeks, a prompt referral to a GI specialist for further workup such as endoscopy is in order. The clinical symptoms vary depending on the area of the gastrointestinal tract affected and can be useful in distinguishing the different EGIDs. Of all the EGIDs, however, eosinophilic esophagitis is by far the most common so we're going to focus on that.

Eosinophilic Esophagitis (EoE)

EoE, briefly described in Part 1, is a relatively new disease that was first documented in 1993 and doctors increasingly gained awareness of it in the early 2000s. Its defining feature is chronic inflammation of the esophagus associated with dense numbers of eosinophils, which are a type of cell. The prevalence of EoE appears to be increasing, with a recent study my colleagues and I published indicating that it affects 1 or 2 in every 1,000 US children and adults. As previously noted, EoE can manifest at any age and occurs more commonly in males than females. In older children and adults, common symptoms include painful swallowing, the sensation of food getting stuck in your throat/neck/chest, heartburn, and chest pain with swallowing; in younger children and infants, refluxlike symptoms, vomiting, abdominal pain, food refusal, and failure to thrive are the most common symptoms. In adults and children, chronic cough with meals is surprisingly common. Additional subtle symptoms could include longer mealtimes, food pocketing in the mouth, excess fluids and drinking to wash down solids, and excess chewing or storing of foods in the mouth before swallowing.

When left untreated, the persistent symptoms and chronic inflammation will eventually damage the esophagus and can potentially lead to fibrosis and scarring. Because of the overlapping symptoms EoE shares with other unrelated GI conditions, such as GERD, dyspepsia, celiac, irritable bowel syndrome (IBS, see page 154), and inflammatory bowel disease (IBD), the latter of which includes Crohn's and ulcerative colitis, it's important to properly diagnose EoE before too much damage is done.

The good news, however, is that EoE can be diagnosed relatively easily with an endoscopy procedure to examine the state of the esophagus and look for those characteristic eosinophils (a type of white blood cell) via biopsy. Currently, the primary way to determine what's actually causing the EoE is to embark on an elimination diet to rule out suspects. These food elimination diets (FEDs) have evolved over the last decade or so. Initial elimination diets included six foods often associated with EoE: cow's milk, soy, wheat, egg, peanut/tree nuts, and seafood. The patient will reintroduce these foods one at a time and, at each juncture, undergo an endoscopic evaluation to pinpoint the offending allergen, which then informs long-term dietary therapy. A tiered approach is often used for reintroduction.

Finally, for those patients who can't undergo multiple endoscopies, a single food elimination diet of milk can be tried for three to six weeks with close monitoring of symptoms. If this fails to resolve symptoms, then the addition of four food elimination diets to include eggs, wheat, and soy can also be tried. Again, close monitoring of symptoms and signs will help determine the next steps in management. Food allergy testing by your allergist may determine targeted foods to consider adding into elimination diets.

Dr. Joshua Wechsler is one of my go-to doctors and research scientists in the EoE space. In addition to his work in pediatrics, allergy, and immunology at Northwestern University Feinberg School of Medicine, his specialty includes gastroenterology, hepatology, and nutrition with a focus on broadening the research for EoE. He's quick to point out that EoE is unlike other food allergies. "Not all food allergies are created equal. For me, food allergy is IgE-mediated. When it comes to EoE, food allergy is uniquely different from that disease. It's an organ-specific disease—you only get inflammation in your esophagus. We typically find one to three foods where they are causative of the inflammation. And once you keep those foods out of your diet, the esophagus will normalize. Few people have to stay away from many foods."

More than half the time, in adults with EoE, a scar is found. Those with scar tissue can sometimes be treated with dilation tools (e.g., endoscopic balloons) to open up the space a little bit more to ease with swallowing (this is not serious surgery; a doctor can perform it as part of a sedated endoscopy). In the 1980s and '90s, EoE was often treated as acid reflux, but patients on maximum acid reflux meds did not get better. It's now thought that genetics increase a patient's susceptibility and then something in the environment triggers EoE; in twin studies, only about 40 percent of identical twins share the disease. Risk factors currently under study include early life exposure to acid reflux, antibiotics, and having allergies. When Dr. Wechsler treats patients, he takes a systematic approach so he can keep quality of life a priority; "I want to perform as few scopes as possible and narrow a therapy as possible. Sometimes it's as simple as taking away dairy, but then later they can consume cooked milk (e.g., muffins) and cheese (e.g., pizza)." Improved methods of diagnosis, including transnasal endoscopy, are starting to be developed and utilized.

A NOTE OF CAUTION

With the proliferation of at-home DNA test kits where you spit into a tube and send your genetic specimen off for sequencing, many people might begin to think every at-home testing kit is as precise and accurate an endeavor. But this is not the case with at-home food sensitivity kits. Testing for some intolerances, such as trouble with lactose, fructose, and other sugars, including sugar alcohols (e.g., sorbitol) can be pretty straightforward with breath tests that measure the amount of certain gasses (e.g., methane, hydrogen); abnormal bacterial overgrowth in the small intestine—a sign of gut dysbiosis—can also be determined by some of these breath tests. But most masquerading intolerances are not easily diagnosed and require careful consideration of medical history and diet. Eliminating foods you think are problematic is usually a great place to start.

Gustatory Rhinitis

Have you ever eaten spicy foods and had a runny nose? This common reaction is called gustatory rhinitis (rhinitis is inflammation of the lining of the nose). This is a form of "nonallergic" rhinitis that can be present with various foods ranging from hot chile peppers to bread. Occasionally, sneezing and watery eyes can also occur with this form of rhinitis. The symptoms usually are self-limiting and resolve soon after eating. This type of reaction is not immune based and skin testing will be negative to foods. Eating activates nasal receptors that triggers neural pathways that result in clear glandular secretions. Gustatory rhinitis cannot be treated with oral antihistamines as they are ineffective for this type of rhinitis. Several prescription nasal sprays, such as ipratropium bromide, and topical nasal steroids are effective in alleviating symptoms.

Auriculotemporal Syndrome

Auriculotemporal syndrome, also known as Frye's syndrome, is a nonallergic reaction that occurs after eating and shows up as a localized facial rash. The emergence of the rash while eating can be commonly mistaken for a food allergy. Auriculotemporal syndrome is caused by injury to a nerve, called the auriculotemporal nerve, typically after surgical trauma to the parotid gland or other unknown mechanisms. The syndrome can happen in children with no preceding trauma or injury. Typical signs are a flushed/red rash that occurs in the same location in the absence of other food allergy symptoms (vomiting, hives, swelling, and diarrhea). The rash/flushing disappears quickly and occurs with a variety of unrelated foods. It is important to recognize this syndrome since this rash can occur during feeding infants and young children new foods. The timing of the rash, any associated symptoms, and photo documentation of the rash will help your physician determine the diagnosis. Skin testing and other food allergy workup will be negative. No specific therapy is recommended since auriculotemporal syndrome appears to be a harmless condition with a good chance of spontaneous remission in children.

OTHER MASQUERADERS
Irritable Bowel Syndrome

Irritable bowel syndrome (IBS) is a common gastrointestinal disorder that affects between 10 to 15 percent of adults and adolescents. Unlike its kissing cousin—irritable bowel disease (IBD) that physically damages the gut and is therefore considered a structural disease—IBS is a *functional* disorder without physical damage so you cannot "see" anything with testing. (And people with IBS are more likely to have other functional disorders, such as fibromyalgia or chronic fatigue syndrome.) IBD on the other hand is more easily diagnosed using a combination of endoscopy (for Crohn's disease) or colonoscopy (for ulcerative colitis) and imaging studies, such as contrast radiography, magnetic resonance imaging (MRI), or computed tomography (CT).

The definition of IBS is recurrent abdominal pain that, on average, is one day per week in the last three months and can include diarrhea, constipation, altered bowel habits, cramping, gas, bloating, and mucus stools. As I briefly detailed in Part 1, and per the Mayo Clinic, the precise cause for IBS isn't known, but could include such factors as muscle contractions in the intestines; abnormalities in the nerves in the digestive system, gastroenteritis, bacteria, bacterial overgrowth, or a virus; early life stress; or changes in gut microbes. Triggers for IBS may include breads and cereals made with refined gains (not whole), processed foods, high-protein diets, and dairy (especially cheese). If symptoms are mild to moderate, then education and reassurance along with dietary modifications may be sufficient. Dietary changes may include low-FODMAP diets, gluten avoidance, and high-fiber diets to keep food moving through digestion. Increasing physical activity also can help. More moderate to severe cases may require drug therapy with laxatives, antidiarrheal agents, and antispasmodic therapies. Additional treatments have included biofeedback, cognitive behavioral therapy, and brief psychotherapy. People with IBD can also benefit from dietary modifications but they often need additional prescriptions in the form of drugs that help control the damaging inflammation.

Celiac Disease and Gluten Intolerance

My good friend and a pediatrician in Seattle, Washington, learned about her celiac in a bit of a roundabout way. Her sister had been anemic for years with poor response to taking iron. Her sister's astute primary care physician decided to screen her sister for celiac disease even though she did not have any of the classic GI symptoms, and she was diagnosed by biopsy. Around that time, my colleague's son, who was twelve, was being monitored for poor growth in height. When her sister was diagnosed, it occurred to her that she should test her son. He had a very high tTG level, an antibody indicative of celiac, and was diagnosed with celiac by biopsy as well. They then proceeded to screen all of my friend's close family members. Shockingly, my colleague, too, was diagnosed with celiac. Knowing that they all had intestinal damage and were at risk for various complications, they have learned and adopted how to maintain a healthy, gluten-free lifestyle. Her sister's anemia has resolved, and her son's growth has improved significantly since going gluten-free.

Screening for celiac disease is recommended in patients with symptoms that are consistent with gluten intolerance. In addition, certain high-risk groups should also be screened regardless. These may include people with close (first-degree) relatives who have celiac disease or other conditions that raise the risk of celiac—autoimmune thyroiditis, type 1 diabetes, autoimmune liver disease, Down syndrome, selective immunoglobulin A (IgA) deficiency, Turner syndrome, Williams syndrome, or juvenile chronic arthritis.

The first tests that should be performed are blood tests to include IgA levels and tissue transglutaminase (tTG-IGA). This test is highly specific, sensitive, and more cost effective than other antibody tests. If the IgA is normal but tTG-IGA is abnormal, then an intestinal biopsy will be required. Additional testing could include looking for particular antibody substances in the blood indicative of celiac, such as antiendomysial antibodies, deamidated gliadin peptides, antigliadin antibodies, and antireticulin antibodies. As with any testing procedures, false negative and false positive results can occur. Additional genetic testing and intestinal biopsy may confirm the diagnosis and treatment recommendations. I realize I'm mentioning a lot of technical terms here, but gaining the right vocabulary can help you further understand what's happening with your testing and diagnosis. As always, discussions with your primary care provider and gastroenterology specialists can determine what testing and diagnostic procedures are indicated.

Testing for gluten intolerance in the absence of celiac, what's also known as nonceliac gluten sensitivity, is a bit trickier because there are no blood tests to make this definitive diagnosis that may affect as many as eighteen million people in the US. The actual number of people with gluten intolerance is unknown because there is no diagnostic test for it. The diagnosis is made by exclusion: an individual is first tested for celiac disease and wheat allergy, and if those tests are negative yet the person continues to get ill from consuming gluten, the person is then consid ered gluten intolerant. I should remind you, however, that people who think they are reacting to gluten, and don't have celiac, may actually be reacting to other components of wheat.

Gastroesophageal Reflux Disease

Gastroesophageal reflux disease (GERD) develops when the "reflux" of stomach acid enters into the esophagus and causes troublesome symp-toms, what some call heartburn though it has nothing to do with the heart. The disease is very common and estimated lifetime prevalence is 25 to 35 percent in the US population. GERD is usually diagnosed on clinical symptoms alone; however; some patients may require endo-scopy to confirm the diagnosis. The classic symptoms consist of a burn-ing sensation in the throat, acid taste in the mouth, difficulty swallowing, and at times chest pain. Treatment is usually initiated with dietary edits to eliminate triggers (e.g., caffeine, spicy food, carbonated beverages), and certain medications, such as histamine 2 receptor antagonists (e.g., Pepcid, Zantac) and proton pump inhibitors (e.g., Prilosec, Nexium). Intractable or relapsing cases may require prolonged therapy and refer-ral to a GI specialist.

Hiatal Hernia

Hiatal hernia occurs when the upper part of the stomach bulges through an opening in the diaphragm and into the chest cavity. Symptoms are very similar to GERD, but patients with hiatal hernia can have "attacks" depending on the type of hernia that is found. The most common type diagnosed in 95 percent of cases is called a sliding hiatal hernia. Diagnosis is usually by barium swallow and/or endoscopy. Treatment again is usu-ally by lifestyle changes (weight loss and dietary restrictions of caffeine, spicy foods, etc.), proton pump inhibitors, and in some cases surgery.

MORE MASQUERADERS

Without tossing you the proverbial kitchen sink, let me share a few other less common masqueraders: esophagitis, gastritis, intestinal motility disorders, infections of both bacterial and viral origin, diverticulitis, eating disorders, some cancers, vocal cord dysfunction, and factitious disorder (pretending to be sick).

MASTER MASQUERADERS: NON-IGE-MEDIATED FOOD ALLERGY

Currently there are no validated tests to confirm non-IgE-mediated food allergy, which makes these types of food allergies the more challenging ones to diagnose. These masqueraders primarily affect the gastrointestinal tract and almost always affect children. Non-IgE-mediated reactions are usually delayed and symptoms are generally observed after one hour to days after ingestion of the suspected allergen.

As I've already defined, they do not involve the production of IgE. Well-recognized non-IgE-mediated gastrointestinal food allergies include food protein–induced enterocolitis syndrome (FPIES), food protein–induced allergic proctocolitis (FPIAP), and food protein enteropathy (FPE). These are not common and typically begin in infancy; here's a quick rundown:

FPIES

Food protein–induced enterocolitis syndrome first shows up in infancy with the most common triggers being cow's milk and soy milk, but other foods, such as grains (predominantly rice), meats, vegetables, and fruits have also been reported to cause the disease. Symptoms may be acute or chronic, with acute FPIES being the most common form of the disease. FPIES usually develops in infants under nine months of age. Symptoms occur one to four hours following food ingestion and reactions are quite dramatic. Diagnosis of FPIES is challenging and misdiagnosis is common. Diagnosis of FPIES is commonly based on history alone, absence of symptoms after food elimination, and if necessary, a clinically supervised oral food challenge. In extremely rare cases, FPIES has developed in older children or adults as a reaction to shellfish. Your allergist may often perform additional skin prick tests to ensure that an underlying food allergy doesn't exist as well. It's not uncommon to have FPIES in the clinical setting of IgE-mediated food allergy. In fact our team recently published an estimate that approximately 1 in every 200 US children and 1 in 450 US adults have physician-diagnosed FPIES. However, among children and adults with a current food allergy, FPIES is much more common, affecting an estimated 1 in 25 children and 1 in 115 adults.

FPIAP

Food protein–induced allergic proctocolitis, as previously described, is a non-IgE-mediated food allergy that's a common cause of rectal bleeding in infants. Inflammation in the colon and rectum and presence of blood and mucus in the stools is observed in infants with FPIAP. The most common trigger is cow's milk, followed by egg, soy, and corn. It's seen in both breastfed and formula-fed infants. The diagnosis of FPIAP is based on clinical history and resolution of symptoms following elimination of problematic foods.

FPE

Food protein enteropathy is sometimes referred to as cow's milk–sensitive enteropathy ("enteropathy" simply means a disease of the small intestine). In most cases, cow's milk causes injury to the lining of the small intestine and the most prominent symptom is diarrhea within a few weeks of introducing cow's milk to an infant. Other food proteins, such as soybean, wheat, and egg, have also been implicated in FPE, but again this condition is rare, and by some measures, on the decline.

HOW MUCH WILL THIS COST?

Before embarking on any allergy testing, it helps to have a clear sense of what your insurance will cover, from the allergist ordering the tests to the tests themselves. You'll want to know what you're responsible for out-of-pocket given your deductible, copay, and whether your doctor is in your network. Exactly which tests are ordered, how many allergens are tested, and which labs are charged with providing results all factor into the equation. What you will pay depends on your insurance plan and the relationship between your insurer and your doctor (which is why working with a doctor who does this routinely is key, as they will be able to know from experience what your financial responsibilities are likely to be). Transparency is what you're looking for, so you don't get hit with surprising bills. Again, I should caution you on buying over-the-counter kits sold online. Although their price tag may be enticing, they can send you down the wrong path and you will not have the guidance or supervision of a trained allergist to help you navigate this confusing area. I realize that our health-care system in general can be ambiguous and disconcerting, letting us down when we need it most and sending medical bills we didn't expect. But my hope is that more advocacy in this area will improve the system and remove barriers to people desperate for proper diagnostics who may think they cannot afford proper testing. Reform also needs to happen to close the gap between financially unfit and fit families who have greater access to the best treatments and allergen-free foods and those who do not.

Indeed, living with food allergies can be an expensive endeavor. In fact, back in 2013, my long-time colleague Dr. Lucy Bilaver and I estimated that in the US childhood food allergies cost families approximately $25 billion a year. She and I are currently conducting a follow-up study aiming to better understand the economic burden that food allergies currently impose—not only on families of children with food allergies, but also on adult food allergy patients. This study is particularly important since it will help us better understand and address the socioeconomic disparities that we have observed in our previous studies. These emerging data suggest that food allergies are more frequent, severe, and burdensome among Black and Latinx families in the US. Furthermore, for low-income families, who are often under-/uninsured, life with food conditions can be particularly challenging given the high cost of medications, specialty care, and other necessary accommodations—specifically, allergen-free foods. Our data have repeatedly shown that children with food allergy are less likely to receive an appropriate physician-diagnosis if they live in lower-income households—highlighting the need to improve equity in food allergy management and outcomes.

Emily Brown is founder and CEO of the Food Equality Initiative (FEI), the nation's leading organization working to increase access to allergy-friendly and gluten-free foods to individuals who need them the most. Without her family's struggles with multiple food allergies, FEI would have never come to fruition. Emily learned her daughter was allergic to peanut, egg, dairy, wheat, and soy when her child had an anaphylactic reaction at the age of one to peanut butter. Once learning of her daughter's allergies, they had to make many changes to her diet. Emily, a former preschool teacher, and her husband, a social worker, quickly became overwhelmed with the cost of the allergen-free foods. They realized that there is no safety net for low-income people diagnosed with food allergies or celiac disease. Although she'd planned to go back to work after her daughter turned one, it was too difficult, given her medical needs. And then her second daughter was born with not only food allergy but EoE that took years to diagnose.

Luckily, the EoE diagnosis led to proper treatment with dietary edits and steroids, and a return to thriving as a child. Emily then trained her efforts on education, advocacy, and health equity with the founding of the Kansas City–based Food Equality Initiative in 2014. Emily's story brings to light the challenges of living with food allergy and related conditions that have a tremendous impact on an entire family's financial health and wellness. Food allergy is on the rise but so is the disparity in the diagnosing and treatment of the conditions. Such rare conditions as EoE demand more education and awareness among not only patients and families but also doctors and primary care physicians.

The Value of Retesting and Second Opinions

My colleague Dr. Sai Nimmagadda has been practicing allergy in the Chicagoland area for the past twenty-five years. His interest in allergic diseases developed while he was a research assistant at National Jewish Health in Colorado where Dr. Allan Bock conducted his pioneering work decades ago. He went on to complete his fellowship in allergy and immunology in the mid-1990s and has seen the "explosion of food allergy" in his practice and after he joined the Division of Allergy and Immunology at Lurie Children's Medical Center. Ironically, his son had severe milk and soy allergy that was initially diagnosed as "colic." It wasn't until he had anaphylaxis to milk that the diagnosis was made at around 7 months of age. His son was enrolled in one of the initial milk allergy studies under Dr. Bock. Dr. Nimmagadda tells an interesting story of how his son's oral milk challenge failed at three years of age; then at three years ten months, he was able to tolerate a whole serving of cow's milk with no reactions. It's this personal experience that has formed his passion for encouraging regular allergy follow-up.

During his training at National Jewish Health he learned the value of independent medical assessments. Through the years, he would see numerous patients who were misdiagnosed and patients who "outgrew" their food allergy but were never tested or challenged. During these consultations he would note that testing wasn't repeated in years or noted some flaws in the procedures or test results. At a minimum, he recommends annual reevaluation of all implicated foods, and repeated testing, depending on the food allergens in question. Fifty to 80 percent of the time, infants and children can outgrow milk, egg, wheat, and soy allergy. Around 60 percent of the time, oral tolerance is achieved by the age of six. Allergies to peanuts, tree nuts, and shellfish are significantly less likely to be outgrown, with rates around 20 percent. On the other hand, oral tolerance can develop at any age so constant reevaluation is necessary. This, of course, includes adults who live with food allergy, whether they've had them since childhood or develop them as an adult. They may not outgrow their food allergy, but reevaluating every couple of years is recommended.

Now that you have an idea about your diagnosis or your child's diagnosis, when should you seek a second opinion? Popular to contrary belief, seeking a second opinion doesn't mean that you don't trust your current provider. It is imperative that you get an accurate diagnosis, since a food allergy may mean a lifetime of food avoidance or extended treatment measures. I realize that finding a physician can be difficult, especially if you live in an area where your options are limited and tracking down the ideal doctor may require some traveling. You need someone with who you feel comfortable and can communicate effectively. Sometimes the physician-patient relationship is like dating. You just need to find the right fit for you. Referrals from friends or local support groups often are a good first start to find a qualified allergist. Additional resources could include medical staff at local hospitals in your area. Because of the inherent variability in testing, I would always recommend that you "know your numbers" for both skin testing and any IgE blood tests and CRD results, since these are important values to have when seeking a second opinion.

Reassessing every year or two allows for accurate food allergy diagnosis and discovering the possibility of achieving oral tolerance. Between these visits, you should record any reactions to food (or lack of reactions in some instances), take pictures, and note any treatments given. These accidental food exposures will help in determining what testing is required on an annual basis. Forming a partnership with your primary care doctor and allergist will give you the confidence that you've explored all treatment options and are obtaining the best care possible. Annual visits with an allergist experienced in food allergy provide an opportunity to review issues individual to your needs, education about managing food allergy life, and new information as research unfolds new strategies for care.

I'm Not "Allergic," but I Still Have Symptoms . . . So, Now What?

Okay, let's say you've gone through the process of being evaluated for food allergies across the usual end of the spectrum that involves immunological, IgE reactions in the body. You've even been tested for mixed IgE conditions and some of the rarer disorders, including those that can be serious digestive diseases, but nothing turns up positive. You are convinced you are sensitive to a litany of foods and have restricted your food options to the point you're probably nutrient-deficient and the whole prospect of eating is unpleasant. You've kept rigorous food journals, you've tried every diet, you've ordered genomic testing, and you've even seen a therapist for your anxiety and mood, thinking maybe it's all in your head (and perhaps it's been suggested that it's indeed "all in your head" and you just need a therapist). You haven't felt like yourself in a long time and suffer from unrelenting bloating, gas, fluctuating diarrhea or constipation, fatigue, unexplained nausea, persistent headaches, brain fog, and/or mysterious transient body pain. You're convinced that you're intolerant to most everything. You don't know what to do and would love someone to hand you a piece of paper that definitively tells you exactly what ingredients to avoid. You're not only exasperated by the daily fear and fight with food, but you're frustrated by the lack of quick, easy answers.

And it doesn't help that friends tell you about alternative sensitivity tests on the market that are "proven" to get to the bottom of your food issues. Some of the names of these tests sound compelling and revolutionary: cytotoxic assay tests, hair analysis testing, mediator release assay (a patented test). I won't even go into the details of these tests because they lack the kind of data and evidence-based proof from clinical trials to endorse them. Although they may reduce some guesswork and give you a greater sense of control over your life (because, after all, you're doing *something* to get to the bottom of your ailments), all of these commercial products have limitations and flaws, and many are medically dubious. Moreover, because there's a lack of standardization across different labs, their accuracy may vary by lab. These tests haven't been compared against one another in well-controlled, published studies, so it's uncertain whether one test is better than another. They are not recommended by professional medical organizations, and while they may advertise themselves as being "laboratory-developed," they are not regulated by the Food and Drug Administration. Insurance companies will not cover them. Yet they can be incredibly seductive with aggressive marketing campaigns, preying on desperate people willing to throw a lot of money at these products.

My advice is to be persistent and keep pursuing a proper diagnosis, seeking additional opinions whenever possible. Be sure you're working with a board-certified allergist/immunologist (if you haven't already) with a long track record and bring in support expertise in the form of a gastroenterologist and dietitian-nutritionist who specializes in food allergy or gastrointestinal issues. They may refer you to a rheumatologist or endocrinologist if needed. From there, these experts can recommend further professionals to bring into your sphere. The good news is you can rest assured that you don't have any IgE-mediated food allergies that can be life-threating. Now, the problem-solving turns to all the other possibilities across the other end of the spectrum, and this may even involve some investigative work outside the spectrum entirely with other masquerading health conditions, such as problems with your endocrinology (hormonal system) and such organs as your thyroid (which controls a lot of your body's hormones).

Again, this is why it's important to obtain the wisdom of a health-care professional experienced in this tricky endeavor and who will listen to you and your symptoms. And they will be much more helpful and effective than anything you find online in the DIY department. An elimination diet followed by methodically trying eliminated foods one by one after a period of avoidance is the best way to identify food intolerances. But doing this experiment on yourself is one you'll want guidance on, with experienced practitioners who will track and follow up with you until you have your answers. Use the guide in this book to keep track of your symptoms and take this to your physician to start the discussion. Do not hesitate to obtain a second opinion if you find the need.

REMEMBER TO STOP STOP

As I talked about on page xxviii, a simple acronym to remember and that can guide your path in arriving at solutions to your symptoms is **STOP**:

S: signs and symptoms

+ What are the signs of your food reactions and how would you describe them (e.g., hives, coughing/wheezing, stomach pain, throat tightening, dizziness, vomiting, itchy mouth/lips, other)?

T: type, timing, treatment, and testing

+ What foods do you know cause you problems? What foods do you think may be bothering you? How much do you need to eat of each food to cause a reaction?

+ Is it a single food or mixed with other ingredients?

+ When do your symptoms emerge relative to consuming the food? Within 15 minutes of eating the food, 15 minutes to 2 hours, between 2 and 24 hours, more than 24 hours?

+ What kinds of treatments have you tried, if any? Did you feel better? Any medications?

+ Have you been tested for anything, either on your own or under the supervision of a health-care professional?

O: opinions and options

+ Have any medical professionals offered opinions on your reactions? What type of clinician? What was diagnosed? What
management was recommended?

P: plan and path forward

﹢ Do you have a management plan for your diagnosis?
Medications and/or dietary strategies? What foods are you
avoiding? What treatments work for you?

+ What is your long-term goal? How will you get there?

Remember: Information is power. The more you can track your
experience and document as many details as possible, the more information you have to use in identifying, managing, treating, and
ultimately gaining control of your condition(s) and preventing future
episodes.

Note that many people have a combination of both food allergy
and intolerances that may be difficult to diagnose all under the umbrella of one set of tests or even one doctor. If this describes you, en-
listing the help of a multidisciplinary health center might be key, so it's
much easier to obtain referrals and have a team around you and your
case. Once you've identified immune-based IgE food allergies, you can
then move on to identify other sources of continued physical distress
that could be related to non-immune-based reactions or a disruption
somewhere else in your physiology that mimics and masquerades as a
"food allergy."

Greater awareness and access to diagnostics on the food reaction
spectrum are on the rise, and this could not come at a better time as
there's an explosion of new therapies and treatments. Up next, we're
entering the treatment zone—the most provocative and exciting movement taking place today in food allergy.

Fearless Facts

→ Testing for food allergies and intolerances is far from a precise endeavor with guaranteed diagnoses. Knowing and respecting the limitations of these tests is part of empowering yourself. In many areas of medicine, in fact, tests provide *clues*—not answers. Keep a good history using some of the resources in this book.

→ Masqueraders that are either non-immune based or mixed can complicate matters; there can be overlapping symptoms as well as the possibility that an individual has both classic food allergies and masqueraders.

→ False positives are common: around half of all blood tests of "allergen-specific IgE" levels and skin prick tests can yield a "false positive." A false positive test is one that says you are allergic when you are really not. Testing must always be paired with history.

→ The more clues gathered through lab work, clinical exams, old-fashioned medical history, and, in some cases, food challenges and elimination diets, the easier and quicker it is to arrive at some answers. Tracking your symptoms over time with notes on such details as what you ate and when, and under what circumstances, can provide your physician with key information he or she can use to accurately diagnose your condition. Use the food log in Appendix C as your template for tracking. Remember to STOP:

> **S**: signs and symptoms
> **T**: type, timing, treatment, and testing
> **O**: opinions and options
> **P**: plan and path forward

→ Avoid self-diagnosing with testing kits you can buy online or in the pharmacy. Suspected food allergies should always be evaluated, diagnosed, and treated by a qualified medical professional. Even seeking help with food issues that do not cause serious immune-based reactions should involve the help of medical practitioners and dietitians.

→ It's important to retest with age and changes in physiology as your treating physician sees fit. Also don't hesitate to seek second or third opinions when a diagnosis (or lack thereof) doesn't feel right. When necessary, don't neglect the wisdom of a licensed dietitian and board-certified gastroenterologist in addition to your allergist and primary care physician.

seven

TREATMENT

Current and Cutting-Edge Therapies

S OMETIMES IT CAN TAKE A CENTURY, OR LONGER, FOR AN IDEA TO TAKE flight in medicine from an initial experiment that shows a glimmer of hope. Although it is frequently stated that an average of seventeen years passes by before research evidence reaches clinical practice (what's called translational medicine), in reality, the lag time can be much longer due to a confluence of circumstances, from logistical and technological speedbumps to purely ideological roadblocks that stifle innovation even when an experiment clearly hints at relaying a cure. Such is the case in the narrative about food allergy medicine. Although classic allergic symptoms, such as swelling, rashes, red eyes, runny noses, and short-ness of breath have long been recorded throughout history, dating as far back as ancient China, Egypt, Rome, and Greece (the last was where the word *asthma* originated, meaning "panting"), it was not until the twen-tieth century that advances in immunology finally began to make sense of the full allergy puzzle. Roman poet and philosopher Titus Lucretius Carus famously said in the first century AD, "What is food to one man is bitter poison to others," but no one would define what that meant for centuries.

In 1906, Austrian pediatrician and scientist Clemens von Pirquet first introduced the term "allergy" to mean "altered reactivity." He noticed that patients who had received smallpox vaccinations using horse serum usually had quicker, more severe reactions to second injections. He also noted that some children given antiserum to prevent infectious diseases, such as diphtheria, became suddenly ill. Correctly attributing this reaction to the formation of antibodies and their interaction with specific molecules (called antigens) contained in the serum, he called the collection of symptoms resulting from serum injections "serum sickness," concluding that the reactions, which were similar to the way some people suffered with bee stings, pollen, and foods, were caused by the body overreacting to foreign proteins. Pirquet also used the term "allergy" to describe these antibody-antigen reactions, although his definition—"any form of altered biological reactivity"—was open to much interpretation.

In December that same year, a London doctor, Alfred Schofield, conducted a nifty experiment that would go down in history as the famous "egg poisoning" trial. He treated a thirteen-year-old boy who was allergic to eggs with a daily serving of 1/10,000th of an egg through a pill—a minuscule amount at the start, after which he increased the dosage cautiously until the boy had consumed one whole egg over the course of six months. During that time period, the boy was desensitized from his egg allergy and by eight months, he could eat an entire egg without harm. Schofield documented his achievement for the *Lancet* in 1908, writing that tolerance to even the "most poisonous foods" could happen through "sufficient care and patience."*

You would think such an accomplishment would have made mainstream headlines, provided a beacon of hope to others with food aller-

---

*Ironically, this technique of ingesting minute amounts of a toxic substance actually began centuries earlier (a.k.a. Mithridatism, named after the King of Pontus, an ancient ruler in what is now northeast Turkey) as a way to prevent poisoning by adversaries. The thinking was if you ingested small, nonlethal amounts of a poison, you'd eventually become immune to it.

gies, and marked the beginning of a revolution of sorts in medicine—the first chapter in the story of oral immunotherapy (OIT). Well, it was indeed the first chapter, but the next chapter would take another century to write and the story continues today in clinics and laboratories around the world. Why so long?

Unfortunately, the world—let alone the medical community—was not ready to acknowledge food allergy reactions, which at the time were commonly described as "idiosyncrasies." The observation noted by Schofield was a bit ahead of its time given how doctors thought and had been trained. With no previous experience of, or rich scientific literature, documenting food allergies to provide context and a foundation—not to mention there being a total lack of a universally accepted vocabulary around the condition and its symptoms—many doctors dismissed allergies as a response to emotional stress or neurosis. Even episodes of anaphylaxis were classified by senior physicians as "medical anomalies." With time and the increasing voices from attentive, prescient physicians, that would all change. Food allergy would not be dismissed as "mere fancy" but taken as medical fact, and perceptions would slowly but surely shift.

Breakthroughs in medicine always take time to sink into the con sciousness of professionals steeped in established dogma. As the old saying from Nobel Prize–winning physicist Max Planck goes, and which speaks to the sociology of scientific knowledge: "A new scientific truth does not triumph by convincing its opponents and making them see the light, but rather because its opponents eventually die, and a new generation grows up that is familiar with it. . . . the growing generation is familiarized with the ideas from the beginning: another instance of the fact that the future lies with the youth." This is now known as Planck's principle.

Although plenty of noteworthy physicians had written about food allergy long before there was any medical understanding of the affliction or its relatives on the spectrum—Hippocrates and Galen in the classical period to Ibn Sīnā (980–1037), Thomas Sydenham (1624–1689), and William Cullen (1710–1790)—the field of food allergy remained quiet, undefined, marginalized, and debated. Throughout much of the twentieth century, elimination diets became the diagnostic norm, after which those foods shown to be problematic were simply avoided. Push came to shove, however, when cases of fatal peanut allergy began to emerge in the late 1980s. And because these cases were happening in young children, the phenomenon could no longer be ignored. Things had to change, and change they did. Advocacy for better labeling laws, peanut-free products, and peanut-free zones in public spaces, such as nurseries and schools, launched a new era. As peanut-related reactions and fatalities increased, food allergy research intensified and, eventually, Alfred Schofield's egg poisoning demonstration would have a rebirth. At the same time, noise about other food-related reactions grew in volume throughout the 1990s as people began to use the terms *sensitivities* and *intolerances* loosely (and confusingly). Greater awareness about such conditions as celiac disease and IBS also added new context to the conversation. The spectrum of food-related reactions was well in development and would continue to gain complexity throughout the early 2000s—and begging for clarity by the time I began my work on this book. The work in food allergy would lead the way and eventually address all food-related conditions.

It was in the 1980s that a group of Spanish researchers desensitized nineteen patients with allergies to milk, egg, fish, or oranges. Fourteen years later, a study by the same group had a 100 percent success rate for desensitization, with a control group that saw no change in their allergic reaction. The data flooded in from there. Study after study confirmed that food allergy is a treatable disease. The small but repetitive presence of the enemy wears our defenses down and retrains the immune system. It's like seeing a stranger regularly in your neighborhood; soon enough you're waving hello and engaging in light conversation until one day, you invite them over for coffee or tea.

Once a diagnosis is made for food allergy, treatment therapies are the logical next step. As detailed in the previous chapter, after a doctor has ruled out nonimmunological causes, such as GI reactions to lactose in milk or gluten in wheat or an intolerance to certain food additives (e.g., MSG, nitrates/nitrites), the target becomes treating those allergies that involve the immune system, from relatively benign conditions, such as seasonal hay fever, to the more serious outcomes that land people in ERs gasping for air. And this is when novel therapies in development today come to the fore to Treat.

Due to the volume of information that could flow from covering all forms of possible treatments to every type of food reaction on the spectrum, we're going to focus on the big-bucket topics in this chapter that will address the most common types of food reactions while highlighting the power of immunotherapy. The solution for nonimmunological forms of allergy is typically avoidance of the offender and treating any masquerader, if possible (e.g., using lactose enzyme supplements to consume lactose-containing dairy). New advances are on the way for treating EoE with cutting-edge biologics being tested that could improve current treatment with a dietary protocol and/or doctor-prescribed drug regimen to keep the inflammation at bay. Also for IgE-mediated food allergies, revolutionary help is on the way. And immunotherapy is among the most pathbreaking developments of all in this field.

THE PROMISE OF IMMUNOTHERAPY

Food allergies can upend lives and families. They change how one lives every minute of the day, from choosing what to eat to deciding which social events to attend, how to survive birthdays, barbecues, overnights, large venues like concert halls, theme and ball parks, dinner parties, going out to restaurants, participation in organized sports, and even dating, traveling, and planning to be in unfamiliar settings, or places where you're not in control of the environment, including what's on the table. Buffets, salad bars, ice-cream parlors, corner cafés, food courts at sports arenas or malls, and bakeries are allergenic minefields. Parents with children who have allergies will often go to the moon and back to ensure their kindred's safety, which can mean moving closer to the right health care, taking more time for otherwise simple things such as grocery shopping and meal preparation (adults with food allergy and parents of food allergic children spend 39 percent more time shopping for food than if there is no food-allergic family member), adjusting the budget to accommodate for the added expenses of living with food allergy (the average added cost per child with food allergy is more than $4,000 a year), disrupting their work lives to deal with the health demands of their loved ones when necessary, limiting travel, and even homeschooling kids with severe allergies. It's an endless loop of pondering, planning, worrying, deciding, and dealing.

The prospect of a therapy or cure is incredibly enticing. For most people, however, the goal is not to be able to eat an allergenic food to one's delight someday; most individuals just want to be able to live without the outsized fear of a small, accidental ingestion that triggers a reaction—be it mild and irritating, or acute and life-threatening. It's life-changing to go from enduring unrelenting, chronic fear of food on a daily basis to feeling confident with greater peace of mind that you (and your loved ones) will be okay even if accidentally exposed to a food allergen.

When considering treatments, there are many factors to consider beyond simply how many more milligrams of food protein a patient can safely consume before and after treatment. All the emotional elements that accompany living with food allergy are also involved: anxiety and fear being chief among them. What's more, children with food allergy are at a much higher risk for being bullied; they face being separated from peers at mealtimes in school, being misunderstood and ridiculed, and may not be allowed to play at friends' homes. Families must learn how to manage the uncertainties, unpredictability, limitations, and sheer chronic panic that sets in and that can have serious mental health consequences, including depression. Some surveys show that kids with multiple food allergies, including milk and wheat, are more likely to have lower quality of life, and those with food allergies suffer more with quality of life than do people who are diabetic and rely on insulin medication.

In surveys I've conducted, my team has found that living with food issues can add a lot of extra stress to one's life, including those of others around them. In one of my surveys evaluating the parental toll, for example, on caring for a child with food allergy, two-thirds of parents felt that their child's food allergy affected their own daily lives very much or extremely; one-quarter of parents said that their child's food allergy strained their marriage; and fully two-thirds of caregivers also expressed significant fear that their child would have a severe allergic reaction to food. Despite this fear, the majority of caregivers in these surveys expressed eagerness to enroll their child in a clinical trial for immunotherapy, which as you now know involves giving the child a gradually increasing dose of the food allergen under close supervision in order to train the immune system to tolerate that food. (Only 8 percent of caregivers responded that they would not enroll their child in this type of clinical trial.)

Adults with food allergy likewise have to make the decision whether to treat their condition with such cutting-edge technologies as oral immunotherapy or learn to simply avoid their allergens and be prepared for accidental reactions. They can always revisit their options farther down the road. Besides, the science changes so fast that new therapies will undoubtedly emerge that can be taken advantage of later. That's the one thing I love about my area of medicine: we're not going backward; we'll only continue to develop novel treatments.

We all want to live with a sense of control and agency over our lives and have the freedom to do the things that bring joy and pleasure, eating what we love being among those delights. But when food allergies are part of the picture, quality of life can hang in the balance, like an uninvited guest you can't seem to kick out. Just the thought of using an epinephrine autoinjector needle to treat a serious reaction can foment fear and anxiety in both children and adults. The silver lining, however, is that those scary and disruptive experiences can afford the opportunity to positively cope, as successfully using epinephrine can bring a sense of relief and empowerment after the unknown is faced.

As noted, most food allergy is acquired in the first one to two years of life, whereas the loss of food allergy is a far more variable process, depending on both the individual person and the specific food allergy. For example, whereas most egg allergy is outgrown over time, most allergies to peanuts and tree nuts are never lost. In addition, whereas some children may lose their egg allergy in a matter of a few years, the process may take as long as eight to ten years in other children and may never happen for others. For adults with food allergy that emerges in adulthood, there's rarely a "growing out" of it, though the scientific data is still sorting this fully out. And although clinical trials in immunotherapy seem to focus on children, this technology is being applied to people of all ages today—from nine-month-olds to ninety-year-olds.

Currently, there is only one FDA-approved treatment for food allergy, while several immunotherapy approaches that I'll outline in this chapter are in clinical trials, including those in which the allergen is administered orally, under the tongue, or through a skin patch. While immunotherapy for peanuts is now available on the market, more clinical trials for other allergens such as milk, eggs, and some tree nuts are in the pipeline. Until new therapies or a bona fide cure for food allergies is discovered, oral immunotherapy, while imperfect, is the best intervention we have right now.

One benefit that many patients hope to achieve via oral immunotherapy is improved quality of life. Indeed, emerging data—while limited—suggest that OIT can lessen patient anxiety about food and reduce social and dietary limitations associated with food avoidance. Parents of children who have successfully undergone OIT have reported less stress when their kids are left in the care of others, and don't have to devote as much time to preparing meals. Food allergy patients who are successfully desensitized via OIT can be more psychologically reassured when they eat outside the home, share meals with others, and go on vacation, confidently flying on airplanes, staying overnight at hotels, and visiting foreign locales where the diet may be markedly different than back at home and the presence of allergens can be difficult to ascertain. I should reiterate that not every doctor can perform immunotherapy, and it is not always successful, but the number of allergists around the country using commercial food products to offer OIT as a service in their offices to both children and adults is growing rapidly. And for many people, the treatment is life-changing in ways that are worth the trials and tribulations of going through it. Just ask Susan.

An OIT Story of Triumph

Susan Tatelli experienced her first notable food allergy reaction at thirteen months old. The culprit was a single M&M on Halloween. She turned red in the face, sounded as if she was choking, and then vomited—expelling the button-shaped treat practically whole. Her mother, Caryn, didn't think much about it at the time, and it would take a few more incidences to figure out that her daughter had a food allergy.

It wasn't until Caryn offered her daughter a bite of her chocolate-flavored energy bar in a parking lot in 2006, when Susan was three years old, that the possibility of a food allergy really crystalized. Susan coughed, wheezed, and vomited, motivating Caryn to take action. Doctor-prescribed blood tests soon revealed that Susan indeed had a peanut allergy. She also tested positive to egg. Over the ensuing years, Susan would add tree nuts, soy, and hemp to her list of allergens, the latter of which was hard to nail because it sneaks into a lot of foods without you knowing it. Susan had multiple reactions, and luckily, epinephrine saved the day. Life went on after that and the family made sure to be exceedingly careful. Susan's life had to be micromanaged down to where she ate outside the home, whose house she could visit, and which table she could sit at during lunchtime at school.

As the years passed, Caryn grew increasingly concerned about Susan's future. How would she ever be able to leave the bubble they'd created? What would life be like for Susan as she became more independent?

Could she ever live a "normal" life, or would they live in perpetual fear of the next potentially life-threatening reaction? The call finally came when Susan was eleven years old: she had the opportunity to enter an oral immunotherapy (OIT) clinical trial that happened to be taking place at Lurie Children's Hospital. First, however, she had to qualify. This proved to be difficult because her reactions tended to be delayed by several hours; one night she returned home from the food challenge and found herself using two autoinjectors of epinephrine at one thirty in the morning. It marked the first time she had to self-administer the drug, and it took two tries because her first attempt didn't go so well. But once she got over the hump of effectively using the autoinjector, the experience opened her eyes up to the possibilities. No longer did she fear a reaction so much if she knew she had this tool to help her out quickly and effectively. Large, systematic reviews of studies tell us that despite the struggles endured during these food challenge tests, the ends often justify the means: oral food challenges—irrespective of the outcome—can improve a patient's (and caregiver's) quality of life.

To say Susan's road through OIT was a steep, uphill one is an understatement. She endured a lot of delayed reactions and problems passing the milestones the doctors hoped for. There were a lot of reactions to the dosing up of peanut exposure, and a lot of epinephrine in addition to other drugs along the way—a total of fifteen scary anaphylactic reactions, in fact, while soldiering through the OIT process. At one point, she moved to a private practice where she continued the OIT under a different doctor who tinkered further with her dosing and medications. By her thirteenth birthday, she could tolerate a certain amount of peanuts to the point she no longer worried so much anymore about accidental exposure and gained freedoms that she could only fantasize about years earlier. At fourteen, she passed a twenty-four-peanut challenge that took over two hours. It was like crossing a finish line of an Ironman.

At this writing, Susan is a thriving college student and vocal advocate for food allergy patients. She's starred in our school videos and spoken at our conferences, started a YouTube channel, and even designed an Epinephrine Readiness Training Kit to teach others how to use the device and remove the fear surrounding its use. When asked about how she got through it all, she speaks about grit, hope, mental toughness, and commitment to the uncertainty. "Oral immunotherapy is an opportunity to achieve tolerance, and increased freedom," she says. She can't imagine her life without OIT, and neither can her mom.

One thing that Susan's story illuminates is that every individual must approach OIT with their uniqueness in mind—biologically and psychologically. No two OIT patients are alike in their food allergy experience or treatment. While there are universal patterns and a general framework for OIT, everyone's OIT playbook will read slightly differently, for each person reacts distinctively, reaches their milestones on their own timeline, and may need a support staff of various drugs in addition to the OIT itself to round out the treatment plan. For example, in Susan's case, her fluctuating hormones as she moved through puberty while receiving OIT had an impact that had to be considered in her overall treatment. As mentioned briefly in Part 1, it turns out there can be a relationship between a female's hormonal cycles and the severity of reactions. Susan's hazard zone for having a reaction always seemed to be a few days before her period started.

We as scientists are still trying to figure out the connection between hormones and allergies but what we know so far is that hormones can complicate the picture. Allergic reactions around the menstrual cycle along with the development of food allergies or increased severity after puberty or menopause have been reported. And, as noted, we now have documented allergic reactions in women who respond to their own progesterone during the height of their monthly cycle and that has been categorized as an autoimmune disorder. Autoimmune progesterone dermatitis, as it's called, is not common and is not linked to food, but it reveals the potential connections between allergy and autoimmunity.

Further research will answer questions that remain and help us better understand the relationship between food allergy development and reactions and hormones. Susan's OIT has been "life changing," she admits. Now in the maintenance phase, she takes a prophylactic morning dose of allergens to keep her immune system in shape so it recognizes those miniscule proteins as friends, not foe. It's "exercise" for her immune system. Her reactivity to all nuts, which she eats regularly, has gone down significantly; peanuts are the only thing she has to keep at a certain limited dose. Ten peanuts in the morning and a peanutty snack are her "drugs" today in addition to a few other prescriptions as her support staff. I applaud Susan for being such a warrior and for not giving up. It takes pluck and passion, but what she's achieved is priceless. And she's a statistic of a good, successful sort.

Avoidance Therapy

If immunotherapy is the most aggressive measure one can take today to try to treat a food allergy, then complete avoidance of the allergen is at the other extreme that works for a lot of people. The decision to choose immunotherapy can be a very personal one. In our research and in discussions, I've noticed that caregivers of the youngest children, aged six and under, seem to be the most willing to enroll their child in an immunotherapy clinical trial (in our surveys, more than 60 percent respond yes, and only 4 percent respond no). In contrast, caregivers of children who are thirteen and older are generally least willing to participate, with 44 percent responding yes, and 20 percent responding no.

This makes sense: as children get older and learn to live with their allergy through avoidance altogether, many don't want to undergo the stress of immunotherapy, which is time-consuming and fear-conjuring (especially if there are dreadful memories from previous bad reactions). However, as children get to high school and college and become more independent, there is a new interest and urgency to treat, as they are at the age of wanting to socialize more with friends, a bit more self-conscious and risk taking. Although there are no hard data yet showing how many adults decide to try immunotherapy, my feeling is we'll see more and more adults take the plunge as OIT becomes increasingly available with established, universal guidelines in both academic health settings and doctors in private practice. As with any elective procedure, there will be a mixture of individuals who prefer to go through the process and those who opt out and want to just stick with avoidance. It remains to be seen what percentage of adults will choose one course of action over the other as the therapy gains popularity and a fuller picture of the age-specific risks and anticipated benefits of OIT emerges.

Justin Zaslavsky is one such example of someone who has said "no thanks" so far to immunotherapy and prefers to manage his allergies through traditional avoidance as an adult. Justin has struggled with food allergies all his life, arming himself with two epinephrine autoinjectors and always asking whether there are tree nuts or chickpeas or sesame in anything he eats. He was lucky to grow up with a strong parental support system that allowed him to go about his childhood virtually worry-free, and when he matriculated at Tufts University, he met with the campus dietitian to talk about food on campus so that he could feel safe when eating in dining halls. He thought he had it all under control. And then his first summer during college, while he was working in none other than my lab as a research assistant, a package of kale chips brought to light his hidden secret. I had no idea he had any food allergies. Neither did anyone else in my lab.

The kale chip turned out to be the truth serum, as it contained cashews as a flavoring agent. When his throat began to tingle almost immediately, he ran out and bought Benadryl because he didn't have any epinephrine autoinjectors on him. Back in our research lab, he threw up (a lot) and felt his throat closing tighter and tighter. It turned out to be one of his worst reactions and, barely able to breathe, when we got him to our ER about fifteen minutes later, he needed the equivalent of three epinephrine autoinjectors and three courses of albuterol to open up the airways in his lungs. Ultimately, he was admitted to the hospital.

Justin learned a few lessons that fateful day. He no longer keeps his food allergies secret, and he never forgets to carry his epinephrine autoinjector. He's also become a food allergy awareness advocate. In college, he worked as an EMT, providing epinephrine to patients he could empathize with. He also continued working in our research lab and ended up writing his thesis on data he collected with our team. After graduating in 2019, he completed a policy fellowship in New York City and has since returned to support our important food allergy research, including how to best build education and awareness to all families around food allergies, especially the underserved who do not always have access. Although he'd be a candidate for immunotherapy, it was previously inaccessible to him and he's decided that he much prefers to avoid his allergens than to confront them in that setting and go through the process. But he's totally fine with that decision for now and while he knows he cannot act as cavalier as most twenty-somethings without food allergies, he's living his life to the fullest and understands the potential consequences to his behavior. "Not being neurotic or perpetually anxious is important to me," he says. One benefit that he admits has come out of learning to live with his allergies on his own in young adulthood (without his mother watching over and carrying his autoinjector as she had long done) is he's learned how to cook and has also propelled him toward a career in medicine, research, and policy.

Let me break down for you the options for treating and managing food allergy, starting with the most basic strategy: avoidance. Then, I'll get to the details about immunotherapy and other options soon emerging courtesy of twenty-first-century medicine.

Old Medicine Meets the 21st Century

It comes as no surprise that a guaranteed "treatment" for food allergy is strict avoidance of the allergic food and having emergency treatment (e.g., epinephrine) available for reactions from accidental exposure. It's the oldest solution in the book and will remain that way forever. The decision to take more aggressive steps such as immunotherapy is one that should be made on a case-by-case basis with the person's values, resources, and family dynamics in mind—whether you're a child or adult. This is when having access to allergists who specialize in this area of medicine is key. It's important to have frank conversations about the possibilities—the pros and cons—to the direction you take in treatment, if any. Patients, parents, and caregivers should understand the risks and benefits of each treatment through shared decision making.

Dr. Schofield's experiment at the turn of the twentieth century was not the only early sign that immunotherapy held promising outcomes in treating allergies. A few years after his landmark egg allergy treatment study was published in the *Lancet*, Leonard Noon showed in the same journal that hay fever could be treated by injecting patients with small amounts of grass pollen. His experiments took place in 1911 at St. Mary's Hospital in London (now affiliated with Imperial College London) where Noon was a doctor and maintained a lab; his experiments are considered to be the first successful example of allergen immunotherapy. Although Noon never uses the word "allergy" in his original paper, his discovery marked the beginning of a new era for allergy research and treatment. Sadly, Noon did not live long enough to see the fruits of his labor. He succumbed to pulmonary tuberculosis at the age of thirty-five in 1913. His coworker, however, John Freeman, took up the baton and continued to practice immunotherapy, and in 1930 published the first immunotherapy protocol. William Frankland, a colleague of Freeman, performed the first controlled clinical trial of grass pollen immunotherapy in 1954.

In many ways, modern techniques are similar to those used by Noon one hundred years ago: patients are deliberately exposed to small amounts of the allergen over an extended period and, over time, usually develop a tolerance to the allergen. As these therapies became more sophisticated, they have yielded successful treatments for allergies to pollen, insect stings, pet dander, mold, and dust. Immunotherapy now comes in several forms, including allergy shots (subcutaneous immunotherapy), drops placed under the tongue (sublingual immunotherapy), and ingesting the allergen itself (oral immunotherapy). Although allergy shots for people who are highly sensitive to pollen, insect venom, or pet dander are commonplace today, immunotherapies for food allergies are not nearly as universally established because it's been the greater challenge. Allergy shots are recommended for people with severe or persistent allergy symptoms who do not respond to usual medications. They are useful for those who have significant side effects from their medications. Many people benefit from allergy shots for years after going through a full course of shots. A typical course is at least three to five years. It can take about six months to a year for symptoms to start to subside.

Despite the risks involved with immunotherapies for food allergies, modern technologies are finally allowing us to leverage immunotherapy's power in the food allergy realm. Just as the method is transforming other areas of medicine, chiefly cancer where these therapies are retraining immune systems to search and destroy cancer cells, immunotherapies for food allergies are under rapid investigation and development. Before I get to their different modalities, let's grasp a few important definitions: clinical desensitization, sustained unresponsiveness, and tolerance.

Desensitization is defined as a temporary increase in the dose threshold required to trigger an allergic reaction while receiving active therapy. Desensitization may confer a level of protection in case of accidental ingestion but is usually achieved only after months of therapy and is dependent upon continued treatment. Peanut, egg, and milk OIT have been shown to be the most successful, desensitizing approximately 60 to 80 percent of patients studied. Desensitization rates for other foods have not been as closely studied and some evidence suggests OIT may not be equally successful for every food allergy but I have hope that future studies and therapies will emerge to leverage OIT's power across many food allergies across the spectrum.

The ideal therapy would, of course, be curative and allow an individual to ingest any amount of allergen without symptoms even in the presence of activating factors (such as acute illness or exercise). This is termed *tolerance*, which is thought to be a naturally occurring process. Often when children outgrow their food allergy on their own, we say they developed tolerance. If you need continued allergen exposure to sustain this, it is often referred to as sustained unresponsiveness. This is an active area of research, because we don't know yet all of the biologic mechanisms underlying how a person is truly "weaned" off a food allergy and can continue to tolerate a certain amount of an allergen without routine exposure. It's like keeping a muscle in shape: you need to put pressure and stress on it to keep it strong, but the questions become how much pressure and stress and how often.

Currently, the most studied treatment for food allergy is allergen immunotherapy via three main routes: under the tongue (sublingual), through the skin (epicutaneous), or swallowed directly by the mouth (oral). Treatment regimens consist of daily, incremental doses of whole allergen extracts that are given over the course of months to several years. The overarching goal of immunotherapy is to raise the threshold of an allergen that may cause a reaction. The primary goal is to provide protection against accidental ingestion. We still have so much to learn about how to induce true tolerance and find an actual cure.

Sublingual Immunotherapy (SLIT)

Sublingual is medical speak for "under the tongue." SLIT in food allergies involves giving a small dissolved amount of allergen that's held under the tongue for minutes to promote absorption before being spat out or swallowed. This introduces undigested allergen to cells in the lining of the mouth that promote food tolerance. SLIT doses are increased during an escalation phase until a consistent daily maintenance dose is reached. People usually begin treatment with dosing every two weeks under clinical observation. If the dose is well tolerated, then patients repeat the dose daily at home with dose escalations every two weeks until maintenance dosing is reached.

Some SLIT protocols allow for weekly updosing or increasing amounts and for some updosing to be performed at home, which offers a significant advantage over OIT in decreasing the time and cost associated with frequent clinic visits. Once the maintenance phase is reached, therapy then continues for a period of months to years—it's the training ground for the immune system to hopefully shift gears and become desensitized to the allergen. Although this form of therapy does not seem to elicit as strong an immunologic effect as OIT, possibly due to the limitations of delivering a big dose under the tongue, it's nonetheless showing to be a promising treatment.

To date, SLIT has been used to treat peanut, hazelnut, milk, kiwifruit, and peach allergies. Similar to OIT, some allergists offer SLIT for all food and environmental allergens. In a well-designed clinical trial that involved multiple centers, 14 in 20 people who underwent SLIT for forty-four weeks to treat peanut allergy were able to consume about six peanut kernels or had at least a tenfold increase in the amount of peanut powder they could consume compared to before treatment. These patients were then followed in a long-term extended maintenance phase where SLIT proved to be safe. More than 98 percent of doses were administered without reported side effects, aside from mild tingling and itching in the mouth and throat. No doses of epinephrine were required.

Other studies have confirmed these successful results, though larger clinical trials are still ongoing to try to answer additional questions regarding its use. Some allergists offer SLIT, but it remains an investigational therapy and is not yet widely available. The only forms of SLIT approved by the FDA are tablets for ragweed, such northern pasture grasses as timothy, and dust mites. Tablets used under the tongue boost tolerance to the substance you're allergic to and reduce symptoms. Allergy drops are not FDA-approved and are off-label in the United States. They are not covered by most insurance, including Medicare or Medicaid.

Epicutaneous Immunotherapy (EPIT)

Epicutaneous ("on the skin") immunotherapy—EPIT—was first studied as a method to treat hay fever, but given the increasing prevalence and attention to the treatment of food allergy over the last several decades, efforts have shifted to EPIT for food allergy. As its name suggests, EPIT exposes immune cells in the skin to very small doses of food protein that are on an adhesive skin patch you wear and replace routinely over time. These patches contain a fixed amount of protein in micrograms (μg), but the *length of time* you wear the patch increases; this is notably different than the updosing that occurs in OIT every two weeks under medical supervision until a maintenance dose is achieved. The patch is first applied for 3 hours under medical supervision, and then you wear the patch for 6 hours a day during the first week, followed by 12 hours during the second week, and then from the third week onward, the patch is applied for 24 hours every day. Most people have no problem with the patches, but those who experience skin reactions can be helped with antihistamines or topical corticosteroids.

Patches are being developed to treat peanut, milk, and egg allergies, with the peanut patch currently taking the lead in animal studies and human trials. At this writing, Viaskin Peanut (developed by France-based DBV Technologies) has advanced the farthest in EPIT drug development, having completed the large, Phase 3 clinical trials to test safety and effectiveness in people with peanut allergy, and so far, the results are promising. Positive results have also been reported from a small Phase 2 clinical trial testing the safety and effectiveness of Viaskin Milk in treating patients with cow's milk allergy. In 2019, Children's Hospital of Philadelphia reported that nearly half of kids with milk-induced EoE who were treated with the Viaskin Milk patch for eleven months saw an improvement in their symptoms and, best of all, normalization of their biopsies. This was the first study to look at how the milk patch can help relieve people with the chronic, painful

EoE condition that has no cure. Again, more signs of hope. Viaskin Egg is in preclinical development. (For full updates about where these trials are and new technologies on the market when you read this, go to www.foodwithoutfearbook.com.)

Oral Immunotherapy (OIT)

Finally, we arrive at the most promising grand-daddy therapy of all: oral immunotherapy, whereby people eat increasing doses of their villain to disarm their immune system, effectively retraining their immune system to not pull out all the guns to the problem food when encountered, even in minuscule amounts. As I've already described, OIT has a long history with the earliest account to treat egg allergy published nearly a century ago.

OIT typically starts with very small doses of food allergen consumed under medical supervision. These doses are increased, then increased again, and so on, until a small, tolerated dose is reached that can be taken at home each day. Every one to several weeks, the daily dose is increased, until a maintenance dose is reached that is ingested each day for months or years. Typical OIT doses of food protein are measured in milligrams or grams.

Food allergy patients can access OIT through clinical trials or from allergists in private practice. The food allergies treated with OIT in clinical trials include milk, egg, peanut, tree nut, wheat, soy, and sesame, as well as baked milk and baked egg. (Because the mechanism of action for OIT appears to be the same no matter the food studied, OIT theoretically should work for all IgE-mediated food allergies. But the data so far is strongest in the peanut trials, with wheat coming in second.)

As you've read, the first OIT treatment for peanut allergy received approval from the FDA in 2020. Palforzia, developed by Aimmune Therapeutics and previously known as AR101, is an OIT peanut flour product. Palforzia dosing is standardized, starting at the same small

amount and increasing on the same schedule to a final daily maintenance dose of 300 mg of peanut protein, roughly equal to one peanut
kernel, which is lower than most peanut OIT maintenance doses. In
2020, it was announced that after two years of daily treatment, more
than 80 percent of patients (aged four to seventeen) were successfully
desensitized to 2,000 mg peanut protein (the equivalent of about seven
peanut kernels). Although Palforzia is not yet FDA-approved for adults,
that will likely change and many doctors in private practice have been
using their own versions of OIT for peanut on patients of all ages.
Which raises a good question: How many doctors are treating patients
outside of a clinical trial?

By some estimates, the number of providers in the United States who
offer off-label oral immunotherapy is estimated to be around 2 percent
of board-certified allergists. Dr. Sakina Bajowala, author of *The Food Allergy Fix*, is a board-certified allergist who counts herself among the
many warrior doctors in private practice helping countless allergy sufferers manage and sometimes end their plight. Working in the Chicago
metro area, Dr. Bajowala took on Susan Tatelli's case to continue her OIT
beyond the clinical trial. "This is not new to allergists," she says. "We're
quite good at it." But when she began to establish herself in the food
allergy community as a practitioner of OIT more than ten years ago, she
built the operation from the ground up. At the time, it was said that OIT
should only be done in a research setting, but doctors like Dr. Bajowala
saw an opportunity to push the limits and not just help people stay safe
while living with food allergy but also increase their quality of life. "I
spent a few years researching protocols and modifying them in addition
to my own protocols." There are number of (unstandardized) protocols
but those in the specialty are very collaborative—they share their data,
discuss difficult cases, and establish best practices to promote improvement in the therapy.

Dr. Bajowala treats individuals across all ages, from babies to adults,
and performs multifood OIT routinely (e.g., OIT for peanut, cashew,
and walnut at the same time, or milk and egg together). She admits that

certain ages make for ideal patients. Because the immune system is more malleable in one's developmental years, it can take longer to desensitize an adult. And teenagers can also have issues with compliance. Susan has been among her success stories and she attributes much of it to Susan's bravery, commitment, and selflessness. It was important for Susan to be part of the solution and data for the next generation of food allergy sufferers seeking relief.

Since we know that much of the adversity patients with food allergy (and parents/caregivers) experience is related to ongoing fears around having a very severe allergic reaction if they are accidentally exposed to their allergen(s), increasing attention has been paid recently to developing tools to more accurately measure these "patient-reported outcomes." My close colleagues Drs. Paul Detjen and Manoj Warrier are expert allergists who also treat many patients each month with oral immunotherapy in their private midwestern allergy practices. Over the past year, we have begun developing and testing a new set of questionnaires that aim to assess how the quality of life of immunotherapy patients (and their caregivers) changes as a result of participating in oral immunotherapy. Currently, since most food allergy treatments are not expected to completely cure patients of their allergy; rather, they reduce the potential risks associated with accidental allergen exposure. Therefore, it is especially important that we understand how the day-to-day anxiety and quality of life impairments experienced by food allergy patients are impacted by food allergy treatment.

Dr. Warrier is optimistic and excited about the future of this technology. He's quick to point out that choosing OIT is an individual's choice—just as much as each treatment must be customized to a person's medical profile, needs, and goals, the decision to treat at all is personal. In his words: "While starting the first OIT program in our local community has been the most rewarding part of my medical career, it is important to recognize that OIT is a treatment option that makes sense for some patients and families but not for everyone. It was the right decision for my older daughter with multiple food allergies and for the many patients who have completed it in our practice, but it should not be considered mandatory or the only path to managing food allergies. For many individuals, continuing strict avoidance works perfectly fine."

Dr. Richard Wasserman, medical director of pediatric allergy and immunology at Medical City Children's Hospital and managing partner of Allergy Partners of North Texas, is working to publish much of the OIT data he has compiled from private allergy practices across the country, to better understand the factors associated with patient OIT outcomes. His national network of clinical OIT advisers is currently over four hundred members strong and growing—a display of the increasing popularity of OIT as an emerging food allergy treatment across the US.

Dr. Kari Nadeau, who I briefly introduced in Part 1, echoes these same sentiments. Dr. Nadeau, author of *The End of Food Allergy*, is one of the world's foremost experts on OIT and a leading researcher in clinical trials at the Sean N. Parker Center for Allergy and Asthma Research at Stanford University. Over the past twenty years she's treated thousands of patients of all ages, including a nonagenarian. She has high hopes for not just continued advancements in OIT with better predictive biomarkers but she envisions a lot of potential additional therapies, such as biologics and vaccines. And like me, she's banking on more FDA-approved treatments that will help democratize this area of medicine to make it more accessible to all: "Whatever therapy science delivers, we want to make sure it's available for everybody." And that science will only expand to include a variety of therapies that work together in a biological alchemy of sorts.

Indeed, in the future picture of OIT, there will be more to the protocol than just exposing patients to their allergen in a bid to retrain their immune system. Other drugs will be part of the mix to further make the treatment safer and allow for a quicker up-dosing phase. Some of these "support staff" drugs may include biologics, which are drugs usually made from antibody proteins that attack and interfere with key steps in a biological pathway. They are "biologic" in the sense they are produced from living organisms or contain components of living organisms (they can come from mammals, birds, insects, plants, and even bacteria). Biologics are used throughout medicine to treat a broad range of common and rare diseases and include vaccines, cell and gene therapies, and tissues for transplants. You've probably heard of many of them: Botox, Humira, and Herceptin are all examples. They can be powerful medications and are made of tiny components such as sugars, proteins, or DNA that can be derived from whole cells or tissues.

In the case of food allergy, many biologics being studied right now in clinical trials and are showing promising results. For example, the anti-IgE monoclonal antibody omalizumab (brand name Xolair) and dupilumab (Dupixent) have been shown to block certain inflammatory activities in the body that fuel allergic reactions. In a 2017 study, 83 percent of children receiving OIT plus omalizumab were able to pass an oral food challenge after twenty-eight weeks of multifood OIT, compared to 33 percent of children receiving multifood OIT plus placebo. The omalizumab group also had fewer reactions during OIT. Clinical trials are also ongoing to show whether such biologic drugs as omalizumab or dupilumab can protect patients *independent of* OIT, by raising the threshold for reaction. The hope is these biologics alone can work to raise the bar of one's tolerance to an allergen.

Furthermore, probiotics are also being explored to heighten the immune response and the effectiveness of OIT (more on probiotics coming up in the next chapter). Studies are under way to understand these important additions and whether they are truly enhancing OIT without any side effects.

Without getting into the nitty-gritty details of some other treatments under study, I want to at least mention the possibility of vaccines and transgenic plants joining the arsenal. Vaccines could be designed to positively affect the immune system in ways to divert attention away from allergens and change the immune response. And plants that are genetically engineered to be "hypoallergenic" by tinkering with how their proteins are expressed—essentially deleting or neutralizing the problematic protein that triggers the allergic reaction—could be the foods of the future. But we still don't know yet how altering plants like this will also change other aspects like their taste and texture. Technology is on our side to help us figure this out. Additionally, alternative therapies as stand-alone or complements to such immunotherapies like traditional Chinese medicine (TCM) are currently being studied.

Many questions do remain. Researchers including our lab continue to hunt for reasons that, for instance, someone who is dosing every day to maintain their tolerance to an allergen suddenly and unexpectedly has a reaction. Or why food allergy has reached epidemic proportions in many parts of the world—we have our clues and hypotheses but no definitive answers. Perhaps we may never know the underlying cause(s), and instead must apply our growing arsenal of modern technology toward mitigating, preventing, and treating these conditions as best we can.

We also need to pursue better labeling on food, more FDA-approved treatments to further democratize food allergy treatment so it's accessible to all, and food security. Living with food allergy should not be more expensive than living without it. The Covid-19 pandemic has also driven allergy specialists to ask new questions: Does food allergy affect Covid-19 and does Covid-19 affect food allergy? Because viral infections can affect one's physiology, from damaging organs to altering the immune system indefinitely, more studies need to be done to understand how an illness like Covid-19 can trigger new vulnerabilities across the food reaction spectrum—from classic food allergy to intolerances, gastrointestinal disorders, and everything in between. We also need to figure out how to make sense of some people's allergic-like reactions to certain vaccines against Covid-19. How can we develop hypoallergic vaccines or know who is at most risk for reactions? The pandemic is changing the landscape of our lives. How will it change the landscape of medicine? We like being kept up at night by these questions. There's always something to work on, and it's a privilege to rise to the occasion.

I love how my colleague and friend Dr. Nadeau puts it: "When your patients are your inspiration and you launch a commitment to them, it compels you to keep going."

HOW TO FIND A CLINICAL TRIAL

In addition to following your doctor's lead on accessing clinical trials relevant to your (or your child's) food allergy, a great place to start is at the National Institutes of Health's website that features resources and digital doorways to clinical trials. Go to https://www.nih.gov/health -information/nih-clinical-research-trials-you/taking-bite-out-food -allergy. Not sure whether to go the clinical trial or private route? There are pros and cons to each. Clinical trials are free but there are barriers to entry, such as qualifying to begin with and being able to meet the demands and expectations of the treatment protocol, including the trial's physical location and numerous appointments. As with most factors in these kinds of therapies, individual needs and limitations must be considered and a personalized plan must be designed. Ask questions. Do your homework. Use resources at www.FoodAllergy.org.

Fearless Facts

→ Revolutions in treating food allergy took place in the twentieth century, which were further catalyzed by immunotherapeutic advances in the twenty-first century. This area of medicine will continue to advance rapidly with many promising new food allergy therapies currently under investigation, which ultimately aim to take the fear out of food for everyone.

→ There is now a FDA-approved oral immunotherapy for peanut allergy (i.e., Palforzia) and more are on the way. An increasing number of board-certified allergists and immunologists offer the treatment and follow established protocols.

→ For many food allergy patients, and especially for patients with masqueraders and intolerances, avoiding their trigger ingredient is the ideal path forward to treat and live with their condition.

→ Advances in regulations around labeling of commercial foods will continue, which will hopefully make it easier to spot problematic ingredients and curate your diet.

→ Often, combination treatments are appropriate for people with a mix of food-related conditions, from potentially severe allergies and relatively mild masqueraders to underlying GI ailments usually exacerbated by certain foods.

eight

MANAGE AND PREVENT

Setting the Stage for a Reaction-Free Life

HAVING FOOD ALLERGIES AND INTOLERANCES OR LIVING WITH SOMEONE who has them is complex, and sometimes scary. One minute, you are totally fine and the next, after coming into contact with an allergenic food, a severe, life-threatening reaction could unfold with no way to hit Pause and Reverse. Or you eat something that sends you to the bathroom and bedroom for a day because it has upended your digestive system and triggered a migraine.

Food is an integral part of life. Three meals a day plus regular snacking all bear risks. Then, there are the celebrations, social gatherings, and holidays that revolve around food. It can be very difficult—not to mention stressful—to avoid problematic foods, even though they might appear calm and even-keel. No matter how mild and seemingly innocuous previous reactions have been, at the back of many patients' minds is a profound worry that their next bite could trigger a trip to the emergency room—or worse.

As a doctor and researcher who specializes in food allergy, I know this from talking to hundreds of parents and speaking with adults with new onset allergies and intolerances. But as a mother myself to a

daughter with food allergies, it is part of my daily world and I can empathize with those living with food-related conditions. These personal
and professional experiences inform my clinical and epidemiological
work; in addition to my research on the best practices for preventing
food allergy, I've devoted much of my time and energy to understand
how food allergies impact both families and communities and what we
can do to help mitigate the impact.

Management and prevention go hand in hand. **When you manage,
you prevent. And when you prevent, you manage.** In this chapter, I'll
provide a collection of strategies to cover both territories.

One of the key ways to prevent food allergies is early introduction
of foods to babies, with the majority of research to date having been on
peanut and egg. But new data are emerging on other food allergens as
well including through a large study in our lab. I realize that many who
are reading this book may have already been diagnosed with food allergy
and/or related conditions and are not in need of lessons for the prenatal
and infant periods in life. But some may, however, want to know about
the new guidelines for introduction of food allergens in early life (i.e.,
ideally before one year of age) and it would be neglectful of me not to
include this important information. Feel free to skip over this next section and move on to more practical information about navigating your
world, or come back to this when you're in a position to need these
instructions for yourself or a loved one.

Preventing food allergies and other food-related conditions is on
everyone's mind these days, especially among those who plan to have
children. There's not much evidence yet on how to prevent non-IgE-
mediated food-related conditions, such as intolerance to dairy products
(in the absence of milk allergy), gluten-containing grains (in the absence
of celiac), or intolerance to food chemicals and additives, or caffeine.
These types of food-related conditions, as well as food allergy, likely
spring from a complex array of factors, both genetic and environmental.
Sudden onset of a food intolerance that wreaks havoc on your digestive system (but does not involve the immune system that can lead to

anaphylaxis) and depletes your energy or triggers symptoms such as migraines and fatigue could be the result of underlying genes combined with an event that somehow changes the body, such as an illness or infection. We still do not know why someone may suddenly—at any age—have trouble consuming certain foods or ingredients that had previously been enjoyed.

However, as previously noted, many food intolerances can be managed by avoidance of the food or taking certain supplements to help with digestion; lactose intolerance, for example, can be treated with lactase enzyme supplements or by choosing lactose-free dairy. Similarly, although IgE-mediated food allergies are also known to result from interactions between genes and the environment, there is an emerging scientific consensus around ways we can reduce the risk of these more serious reactions. As you might have guessed, this starts at the very beginning of a child's life, when food is first introduced.

EARLY LIFE: LEAP ON!

Socrates, the first moral philosopher and founder of Western ethical thought in classical Greece, may not have had food allergies, but he will be forever attached to the condition. He was often called ἀτοπία, which means "out of place" or "different." More than two millennia later, the term *atopy* (derived from ἀτοπία) was used to describe the atopic family of diseases: atopic dermatitis (eczema), food allergy, asthma, and hay fever (allergic rhinitis, or seasonal allergies from grass, weed, and tree pollens).

As you've learned, the relationship between allergic diseases and progression from eczema/food allergies to asthma and hay fever is characterized as the "atopic march." It's also sometimes called the "allergic march." In fact, studies have shown that two-thirds of patients with eczema develop hay fever and one-third develop asthma. Asthma attacks can be ignited by things as diverse as cockroaches, dust mites, cigarette smoke, or environmental pollution due to living by a highway or power station.

Often, the first sign of allergic disease is eczema, occurring during infancy or early childhood. It is found in 10 to 20 percent of all children. Breaks in the skin's barrier early in life literally open the door to irritants that can compromise a delicate, developing immune system. Food allergies also tend to develop early in life; a child who experiences this "march" is at much greater risk for developing food allergies. The atopic march is driven by both genetic and environmental factors, and though these conditions often start in childhood, this succession of diseases can happen later in life. As I have also already covered, some children outgrow their allergies and have fewer asthma symptoms and some develop asthma and allergies for the first time in adulthood.

Although predicting exactly which children will go on to develop these conditions has been difficult, new findings published in the *Journal of Allergy and Clinical Immunology* have shown just how highly correlated these allergic conditions are during infancy and early childhood. The findings stem from the Canadian Healthy Infant Longitudinal Development (CHILD) Study, a birth cohort study following 3,500 Canadian families and their children to help determine the root causes of such chronic diseases as asthma and allergies, among other conditions. When researchers analyzed the records of 2,311 children enrolled in CHILD, they came to the following conclusions: One-year-old infants at most risk for developing asthma by the time they turned three had both eczema and allergic sensitization. The most common foods they were sensitized to were egg white, followed by peanut and cow's milk. Babies who did not show sensitization to food allergens, but who had eczema, were not at increased risk of asthma. The heightened risk for allergic diseases among those children with eczema and allergic sensitization was significant: seven times more likely to develop asthma, and twelve times more likely to be diagnosed with hay fever. They also carried a much greater risk for food allergy. Bottom line: the combination of eczema with allergic sensitization at age one *predicts* children who are more likely to have asthma and food allergy.

The moment a woman attempts to become pregnant with a child of her own, she (and probably her partner) devours any information to know what—and what not—to do to ensure a safe and normal pregnancy. She'll read books on pregnancy, consume everything she can online, join virtual mom groups, and ask many questions to other moms as well as her doctor. There's no shortage of reading material on the dos and don'ts of pregnancy. She'll soon learn that certain foods are a no-no: raw sushi; undercooked, raw, and processed meat; unpasteurized milk and cheese; and alcohol; to name a few top-listed items. But what about foods that could potentially be allergenic to the baby? Ask pregnant women on the street and you'll likely be met with conflicting responses and considerable confusion—which is understandable, given the relatively rapid shift in recommendations over the past two decades.

When the American Academy of Pediatrics modified its guidelines on how to introduce certain foods to babies, which followed Dr. Gideon Lack's seminal work (see Chapter 3), it was not headline news. The update was not even an overnight sensation quickly adopted and enforced by pediatricians. A survey I conducted and published in 2020 showed that while most pediatricians were aware of the new guidelines, less than a third of them were fully implementing them in their practices. And even as I write this in the fall of 2020, there remains a lack of clarity regarding when and how to safely introduce other common allergens during infancy.

Many pregnant and breastfeeding women still avoid peanuts, cow's milk, shellfish, and eggs for fear that exposure will increase the risk of having an allergic child. I should reiterate that no strategy for avoiding food allergy is perfect. Parents shouldn't blame themselves if their children develop food allergies. Despite the very strong effects observed in Dr. Lack's LEAP study proving the importance of exposing kids early to peanuts, some LEAP participants in the intervention group did end up getting peanut allergy despite doing exactly what they were told to do.

In the spring of 2020, FARE—the nonprofit organization dedicated to food allergy awareness and improving the lives of those with food allergies—launched its Baby's First resource (www.babysfirst.org) to help families navigate new data and information concerning early feeding and recommendations of allergy prevention for babies. Many organizations in the US and around the world are working to spread this important information directly to expectant parents and families. A new consensus statement by three major allergy organizations was released in 2021, outlining additional recommendations (see Appendix A).

EAT

A subsequent trial by Dr. Lack's LEAP team entitled EAT (Enquiring About Tolerance) aimed to investigate whether the introduction, from three months of age, of six allergenic foods (milk, peanut, sesame, fish, egg, wheat) into the infant diet, alongside continued breastfeeding, reduced the number of children developing these food allergies and other allergic diseases (such as eczema and asthma) by three years of age. This "early" introduction of allergenic foods alongside breastfeeding was found to be both safe and could help prevent food allergy. Although there were some issues with compliance among parents sticking to the dietary regimen in the study, the results did show a notable reduction in food allergy prevalence among those who consumed sufficient amounts of allergenic foods from three months of age compared to babies whose mothers followed the UK infant feeding advice of exclusive breastfeeding until around six months. Importantly, the study found that introducing these allergens early didn't affect breastfeeding rates, which is great news because the benefits of breastfeeding are well known.

My team is currently at the forefront of food allergy prevention re-search. We are conducting two studies, Intervention to Reduce Early Peanut Allergy in Children (iREACH) and Start Eating Early Diet (SEED), in an effort to reduce food allergy incidence in infants. Through iREACH funded by the National Institute of Allergy and Infectious Diseases (NIAID), we have partnered with over thirty clinics and over two hundred pediatric clinicians in Illinois to implement a clinical decision support (CDS) tool in clinicians' electronic health records to assist them in adhering to the new guidelines here described and help promote best practices surrounding early peanut introduction.

By helping clinicians and families adhere to the early introduction guidelines, we hope to decrease the development of peanut allergy in infants. Additionally, we're launching the SEED clinical trial that aims to expand these guidelines and determine the efficacy of early introduction (specifically of peanut, egg, walnut, cashew, soy, and sesame) to protect against these food allergies. SEED will investigate whether feeding multiple allergenic foods to infants aged four to seven months, depending on risk, can reduce their risk for developing food allergies. These two studies have the potential to reverse the epidemic of food allergy and potentially other atopic conditions.

MANAGE AND PREVENT FROM A PLANETARY PERSPECTIVE

By taking a big picture approach, we can bring the management-prevention juggle into balance. There's a lot we can gain from looking at what we know globally—which food allergies and intolerances in particular are increasing and where? What we can learn about environmental contributors from around the world? There are clues to pick up if we look closely at the patterns of food-related issues in different countries, continents, and under different environmental forces—from basic geography to cultural influences and lifestyle factors. In my work, we found the food allergy prevalence in urban areas is over 10 percent, while in rural areas it is closer to 6 percent. Research suggest farms are protective and factors in urban areas may be harmful. Also, types of food allergies vary by urban or rural environment and also by country. It seems common foods eaten in countries are common allergens. Some examples include hazelnuts being a common allergen in France, with chickpeas a common one in India.

Our collective internal and external environments also must be factored in, for we know that people who live in urban environments are at greater risk for all manner of food-related conditions (as well as cognitive deficits and metabolic disturbances). This is a message for not only urban dwellers but urban planners, government regulators, and even corporate industry. The indoor environment presents a double-edged sword. On one hand, we know that airborne allergens, such as dust mites, pollens, fungi, and animal dander, can contribute to and exacerbate allergies, especially asthma, hay fever, eczema, and contact dermatitis (skin rashes). Chemicals found in household goods, including cosmetics, fragrances, detergents, soaps, and plastics, can also trigger and worsen allergies in sensitive people.

On the other hand, we have to respect the hypothesis that says too much cleanliness can impair our natural immune defenses and lower our threshold for allergic responses. Now, I'm not about to suggest we stop bathing, washing our hands, and practicing good hygiene in the name of public health (especially in the era of Covid). But there's something to be said for promoting safe exposure to a diverse array of microbes and not being so fast to demand prescriptions for antibiotics when we catch a cold. When we oversanitize our living spaces and misuse antibiotics, we could be setting ourselves up for greater risk for allergic conditions. We must strike a chord between promoting good hygiene and letting some "dirt" into our lives to keep our immune system in shape. We also need to engage in habits that bolster the health and function of our resident microbial collaborators too. This is largely accomplished through eating a healthy diet rich in gut-loving fiber and probiotics.

I should point out that despite slick advertising by marketers of "immune booster" products, such as those that fill the largely unregulated vitamin and supplement industry, there's no such thing as an immune-boosting pill, powder, bar, shake, juice, elixir, potion, or food. The best immune boosters are the habits we keep to support the body's innate defenses: a nutritious, diverse diet, regular exercise, restful sleep, managed stress, etc. (see below). To that end, let me present the 5 Ds and the 5 IBs (science-driven immune boosters).

REACTION PREVENTION & MANAGEMENT 101

Keep abreast about environmental issues affecting food allergy by reading data-driven sources. Minimize your carbon footprint by choosing locally grown fresh foods wherever possible, by reducing meat consumption (the meat industry is a contributing factor in the climate change that may fuel allergies), and by being mindful of your hygiene habits. Think about using less toxic, "greener" cleaning products at home; use a vacuum with a HEPA filter and keep air ducts clear with annual maintenance; and stay on top of dust that attracts mites. Dust mites, rodents, and cockroaches are a huge source of indoor allergens that can be controlled. When buying such clothes, fabrics, upholstered furniture, flooring (carpeting, hardwood), and mattresses, aim for products that are as natural as possible and free of stain-resistant and fire-retardant substances. I realize this is not possible in all cases and that's okay. The goal is to minimize the level of environmental chemicals, much of them synthetic, floating in your home that could worsen allergic diseases. Don't drive yourself crazy in these pursuits; take the cleanup of your home one purchase at a time. You don't have to remodel or throw out everything and start over. Remember, too, that there's a lot you can accomplish at filtering out your air just by opening the windows, weather permitting!

The 5 Ds

My colleague Dr. Katie Allen spent much of her career as a doctor and research scientist unraveling the mystery behind the rising food allergy epidemic in the modern world before joining the Australian parliament. She, too, takes it personally because she's a patient herself and carries an EpiPen with her everywhere she goes, in the event she mistakenly ingests peanut. Unlike most people, however, she developed her allergy as an adult after the birth of her first child. I love how she sums up the main strategies ("The 5 Ds") to consider in pursuit of managing and preventing allergies given the facts we know so far about why these conditions develop at any age:

Diet diversity: Don't delay giving potentially allergenic foods to babies until after they turn one year old (see Appendix A for early introduction to food). And avoiding allergenic foods, such as peanut, during pregnancy does not lower risk. As an adult, keep your diet diverse and nutritious.

Barring problematic foods, you would do well to maintain as healthy a diet as possible in addition to keeping it diverse. The typical Western diet, rich in refined grains, sugary beverages, and fatty and processed foods, is suboptimal for promoting immune health. Much to the contrary, such a diet deprives the immune system of the antioxidants and nutrients needed to help it function properly. You also don't help maintain an ideal gut flora (the microbiome) in the GI tract, home to a significant number of immune cells. Remember, a stereotypical Western diet reduces diversity in the gut microbiome and is associated with bad health outcomes, from chronic inflammation (which itself is a lingering activation of the immune system) to an increased risk for chronic diseases across the board, from diabetes and obesity to heart disease and dementia (see next section).

One antidote that many people find quite palatable is a Mediterranean-style diet that contains fresh fruits and vegetables, legumes, nuts and seeds, olive oil, whole grains, and lean proteins (e.g., fish, poultry). Red meat and certain full-fat dairy, such as cheese and ice cream, are limited. Again, allergens and other problematic ingredients must be taken into consideration, but this diet is easily followable with individualized attention to detail. Of course, there are many diets that are healthy and may be right for you. People all over the world have an immune system and microbiome that are somehow used to the foods in their diet; it's when they move to Westernized countries that they tend to develop the diseases of those places faster and could be missing out on some protection from their homeland diet.

And, of course, if you've been diagnosed with a condition that may respond positively to a special diet, such as a low-FODMAP protocol or a wheat- and dairy-free regimen, seek out resources to help you plan meals and make your special diet work for you while also remaining as diverse, delicious, and nutritious as possible. There are plenty of reliable online sites and books to help you in this endeavor. Just be sure to do your homework (due diligence!) and follow the advice from credentialed, well-respected authorities.

Dogs and dribble: Based on the Hygiene Hypothesis, it helps to be exposed to other animals, pets, and even other people. Studies show that having a dog and an older sibling reduces the likelihood of allergies in infants. Remember, the immune system needs to be exposed to appropriate stimulation during development and throughout life so that it is trained and remains in shape to attack things that might cause us harm (e.g., bad bacterial or viral infections) while ignoring harmless substances, such as foods.

Dirt: Also based on the Hygiene Hypothesis, it helps to get dirty once in a while—exposure to microbes that challenge the immune system help train it to act stronger and normally. One study even showed that when babies routinely used pacifiers that had been dropped on the ground and whose parents "cleaned" their pacifier by sucking on those binkies, their risk for allergies was lower. The "dirt" in this situation is the collection of microbes transferred to the child via the parent's saliva, and which stimulates the immune system in a healthy way.

Vitamin D: Dr. Allen's research has found that infants who are vitamin D deficient are three times more likely to have an egg allergy and eleven times more likely to have a peanut allergy. Those with vitamin D deficiency are also more likely to have multiple rather than single food allergies, with the odds increasing to ten times more likely among those with two or more food allergies. More research is needed in this area, however, because defining vitamin D insufficiency and deficiency remains debated, and you can get too much of a good thing: remember, reviews of studies show that vitamin D intake above the recommended amount may increase risk for food allergy. So, mega-dosing is not a good idea. Most of us would do well with more vitamin D in our life from such sources as safe natural sunlight (the kind you get when you're outside, but not in danger of overexposure to increase risk of skin cancer), fortified foods, and doctor-recommended supplementation. Note: Vitamin D toxicity is possible with oversupplementation, so be wise and consult with your doctor before self-dosing through supplements.

Dry skin: Compromised, broken skin—especially early in life and in people who are susceptible to develop eczema—can be a gateway for sensitization to food, so making sure the skin remains moisturized and intact is important.

The 5 IBs (Immune Boosters)

The following tips are sensible for healthy living and will go a long way to help support healthy biology, which in turn plays into risk for disease and any condition across the spectrum. Although there's no direct evidence to link these with reduced reaction outcomes, the immune system is key to everything.

Regular Exercise

Living a sedentary life (i.e., being a couch potato) also does not serve immune function well. We humans evolved to move and move frequently. I know I'm not the first person to tell you this, but it bears repeating. When you avoid routine exercise that gets your heart beating at a faster clip, your blood pumping at a speedier pace, and your skin sweating, you put yourself at higher risk for the same things a Western diet will do: more inflammation and more chronic disease. Exercise, however, is nature's miracle on the body, arguably providing more health benefits than any drug—and with almost no side effects. It reduces risk for all manner of ills, flushes out stress hormones while balancing blood sugar and metabolism in general, improves the health of every organ and system, and may even help elevate the diversity of the gut bacteria.

Although the recommended amount of exercise is 150 minutes a week of moderate-intensity activity (e.g., brisk walking for a little over twenty minutes a day), more is definitely merrier in this department. You don't have to train for an endurance event, but see whether you can maintain a regular routine for at least thirty minutes daily and that, throughout the week, you cover all the bases—cardio, strength training, and stretching for flexibility. There's no excuse today not to, given all the tools online now to leverage, from streaming videos to virtual memberships to live classes. Or, if hiking or strolling your neighborhood is your thing, listen to your favorite podcast and pound it out with some 3-pound weights in your hands. Just moving more throughout the day has benefits. Even low-intensity physical exercise—walking, doing household chores, and standing rather than sitting—has surprisingly positive health benefits.

Note of caution: For some people, rigorous exercise needs to be properly managed if it exacerbates reactions (and for those undergoing

OIT, your treating physician will give specific guidelines). But even for food allergy patients on the strictest of treatment regimens, there are always opportunities to engage in exercise. So, even though you may have to be a little creative and/or plan ahead, exercise is doable and an important part of any healthy lifestyle.

Restful, Restorative Sleep

Sleep is medicine. A compelling influx of scientific data shows how sleep acts as a natural drug (like exercise) to recalibrate our body, reorganize our mind and memory, and refresh our cells and tissues all the way down to the molecular level. Sleep restores our body at every level from the brain down to the cells in our toes. Entire books are written about sleep today (go there for all those details). Prolonged sleep deprivation has been found to decrease immune function, promote inflammation, raise levels of cortisol (a key stress hormone), and increase risk of chronic disease. You might be surprised to know that the number of circulating, policing immune cells actually peaks at night, which says a lot about sleep. A good night's sleep can truly help fix what ails us.

Sleeping well helps balance the hormones that regulate our biology and immune state; it also affects how well we *feel* and cope with daily stressors, how fast our metabolism runs, how robust our brain operates and thinks, and even how our microbiome functions. While it's hard to consider our sleep impacting gut bacteria, new science shows that indeed there are lots of relationships back and forth: a healthy microbial gut community helps us sleep and sleep better, and a good night's sleep nurtures diverse, sanguine colonies. It's a two-way street. Everyone's sleep needs are different. In general, children need more sleep (10 to 12 hours) than adults (7 to 9). Quality, however, beats quantity. You can sleep for nine hours and still feel tired the next day if you haven't banked enough refreshing deep sleep. The key is to have consistent sleep that moves through all the phases at night repeatedly in sync with the body and fosters a healthy sleep-wake cycle and circadian rhythm.

Reducing Chronic Toxic Stress

We all experience stress; it's an inevitability of life and it can be healthy and motivating in many ways. It's the toxic stress, however, that we need to be mindful of and do what we can to minimize it—and its effects. Toxic stress is the kind that's unrelenting, prolonged, and so psychologically troubling that it begins to impact our mood, biology, and ability to cope. When the stress hormones start pumping with no end in sight, lots of things happen in the body, the least of which is the immune system can decline and lose some of its power. Refer back to Chapter 4 for more about stress (and, specifically, its effects on the immune system via the microbiome).

Stress management comes in many forms, from physical actions, such as exercise, meditation, yoga, and deep breathing, to such basic strategies as sustaining a vibrant social life with reliable friends, keeping those good diet and sleep habits, establishing boundaries between work and play, and making time for hobbies. Many books have also been written on this topic alone (see Resources). There's no single solution—you have to find what works for you and that you enjoy doing. For food allergy sufferers, the stress load can be extraheavy on both the patient and family. Do not hesitate to join support groups, both in person and online, and reach out to counselors and therapists when necessary. For some people, coping with the anxiety and fear of food allergy can demand special attention and a new set of skills. You'll find gateways to help at both www.FoodAllergy.org and www.feinberg.northwestern.edu/sites/cfaar/.

Don't Smoke and Reduce Alcohol

These habits need little explanation. Smoking and excessive drinking are immune system sinkers. They are among the most insidious immune-compromisers. While there's room for moderate drinking (one drink per day), there's no room for smoking or vaping. Think about it: When you inhale that poison, you send your immune system to your lungs, sinus passages, mouth, and throat, beleaguering the entire system. Smoking has a long-documented history of compromising the immune system; the more than seven thousand chemical compounds found in cigarette smoke alone can interfere with the immune system. Most diseases are worsened by smoking, and quitting the habit will go a long way to protect your overall health and reduce risk for illness.

Wash Your Hands

The Covid-19 pandemic made us all think about this habit more frequently. And for good reason: it's long been shown to reduce risk of infection and protect the immune system from unwanted invaders that could send the immune system into overdrive. I don't know any patient of mine who enjoys shouldering the weight of living with food allergies or sensitivities *and* a bad infection. Although there's something to be said for challenging the immune system regularly to flex its muscles, so to speak, we'd all do well to avoid the more adversarial pathogens that can result in serious illness.

For many pathogens, especially those for which we have no vaccine or cure, we don't know their long-term effects, including those that impact the immune system. You'll recall I mentioned how certain infections may be fundamental players in the immune dysfunction that in turn can trigger an allergic disease. Future research will help us better understand the connections, and for now the best we can do is dodge the harmful bullets with proper hand washing (and regular physician checkups when possible, see Bonus IB below).

BONUS IB: KEEP UP WITH ANNUAL PHYSICALS

Keeping up with your regular checkups in general is a good overall strategy to ensure you're staying on top of any health issues regardless of those related to allergies and food intolerances. Masqueraders can suddenly emerge that point to food as a cause when in reality, another underlying condition wholly unrelated to food is conspiring against you. Or you may have a masquerader on the spectrum of food-related conditions that requires special attention atypical of classic, IgE-mediated food allergy.

I cannot overemphasize this: The body is incredibly interconnected, sometimes in ways we don't even know about yet. When one system or organ begins to falter, others can take a hit and produce symptoms that will overlap with the myriad food-related conditions I've covered in this book. Even something as simple (and common) as an underactive thyroid, for example, can cause symptoms that seem to be food related, such as constipation, sluggishness, and weight gain. Moreover, evidence is mounting that food-related issues may play into conditions of the thyroid—and vice versa—with the common denominator being inflammation. Celiac disease and hypothyroidism in fact share a relationship, as people with celiac (an autoimmune disease) are at higher risk for a misfiring thyroid. Those annual visits with your general practitioner who will conduct a physical exam and order routine lab work are important. To keep your immune system in check, all systems need to be running smoothly—no smoldering fire or misbehaving happening anywhere.

MINDING THE MICROBIOME

We still have a lot to learn when it comes to our microbial friends that inhabit our insides and outsides. In 2013, the *Canadian Medical Association Journal* stated the facts squarely when a group of researchers referred to the gut microbiota as being a "super organ" with "diverse roles in health and disease." Since then, a multitude of studies have corroborated the importance of a healthy microbiome in the body's overall physiology, from its metabolism to immune function, which in turn factors into risk for health conditions, allergies among them.

The probiotic market has exploded in the past decade. The term *probiotic* is derived from the Latin *pro*, meaning "for," and the Greek word *bios*, meaning "life." Probiotics are the beneficial bacteria you can consume via pill or through such fermented foods as cultured yogurt, cheese, kimchi, or kombucha. Lactic acid fermentation, in fact, is the process by which foods become probiotic, or rich in beneficial bacteria. In this process, good bacteria convert the sugar molecules in the food into lactic acid. In doing so, the bacteria multiply and proliferate. This lactic acid in turn protects the fermented food from being invaded by pathogenic bacteria, because it creates an acidic environment that kills off harmful bacteria. This is why lactic acid fermentation is also used to preserve foods. To make fermented foods today, certain strains of good bacteria, such as *Lactobacillus acidophilus*, are introduced to the sugar-containing foods to kick-start the process. Yogurt, for instance, is easily made by using a starter culture (strains of live active bacteria) and milk. Throughout history, fermented foods have provided probiotic bacteria in the diet.

We don't know yet the ideal composition and species of microbes that make up a healthy microbiome, and studies on the value of taking supplemental probiotics have been mixed. Someday, and given what we know about the relationship between gut health and immune health, our knowledge in this realm may allow us to "prescribe" certain strains of probiotics to help treat or even cure a food allergy or intolerance.

Of the strains that have been demonstrated to positively influence the immune system, species include *L. paracasei*, *L. rhamnosus*, *L. acidophilus*, *L. johnsonii*, *L. fermentum*, *L. reuteri*, *L. plantarum*, and *Bifidobacterium longum* and *B. animalis*. But we are not at the stage yet where these bacteria can be recommended for managing and preventing any food-related condition on the spectrum. Strains in the bifidobacterium and lactobacillus genera are readily available in commercial products, notably fermented foods.

Studies around the world also show that people of different cultures (literally and figuratively) and environments exhibit different microbiomes, so it's hard to say which strains of bacteria are "good" versus "bad." Diversity of microbes seems to be of key importance—the more diverse, the healthier. And there's no better way to consume a rich array of healthy bacteria than to consume them through wholly natural sources, such as sauerkraut, pickles, kimchi, and other fermented vegetables. Once in the gut, these bacteria need to be nurtured by basic lifestyle habits in addition to a good diet, such as regular exercise and restful sleep, which also participate in the well-being of the microbiome. Prebiotics are increasingly talked about too. These are the compounds in certain foods that also promote the growth and activity of beneficial microbes in the gut, but are not in and of themselves microbes. They are types of dietary fiber found in many fruits and vegetables, such as chicory root, Jerusalem artichoke, garlic, onion, leek, banana, asparagus, and dandelion greens (toss those in a salad!).

Earlier I mentioned how cesarean sections may prevent babies from receiving their first "dose" of microbes via their mother's birth canal—a type of "bacterial baptism" that evolved over millennia. Although scientists initially sounded the alarm on this early shortfall, especially given that as many as a third of births today in the US result in C-sections, newer science suggests that the negative effects of this missed baptism can potentially be rectified. Researchers are deep in the process of trying to help us all understand, and potentially replace what's lost among babies delivered via C-sections.

Dr. Maria Gloria Dominguez-Bello of New York University's microbiome project has presented research suggesting that indeed, using gauze to collect a mother's birth-canal bacteria and then imparting them to babies born by C-section by rubbing the gauze over their mouth and nose does help make those babies' bacterial populations more closely resemble vaginally born babies. It's not a substitute for having a vaginal delivery, but it may be better than a sterile C-section and prove an effective therapy routinely done in the future. More research is needed in this area, as well as universal safety protocols for performing this simple procedure that takes minutes. Infant probiotic formulas are also sold that can be added to an infant's diet, but speak with your pediatrician about this possibility should you want to try it, as these supplements are not recommended by any of the international food allergy guidelines. A baby will get beneficial microbes through breast milk and they are often added to formula now too. Research scientists in this area are still teasing out all the details to make more data-defined recommendations.

Antibiotic use obviously can dramatically impact the microbiome, which helps explain why children who receive many rounds of antibiotics early in life (often for chronic infections) go on to live with a higher risk for health challenges, from obesity to allergies. If you're an adult who has lived with health conditions most of your life, food-related issues included, or if you're someone who has developed them more recently, your antibiotic exposure overall could be part of this equation.

Antibiotics are necessary under many circumstances, but they may unintentionally alter the natural bacteria and flora in the intestinal system, which may be enough of a shift in the gut microbiome to alter the immune system—confusing the immune system into triggering allergic pathways. Knowing this evidence can help us try to mitigate their potential damage. Antibiotics play into that Hygiene Hypothesis. Same goes for living in a sanitized urban environment as opposed to a rural area and not having a dander-shedding dog or cat. These settings help maintain a robust and wider array of microbes—all of which keep the immune system in check and help more effectively differentiate between friend and foe.

In 2018, a study in *JAMA Pediatrics* caused a stir in medical circles for its linking the use of acid-suppressive medications during infancy with the subsequent development of allergic diseases, including asthma, in childhood. So, it's not just antibiotics we have to be careful about. And it's not just about kids. In both children and adults, acid-suppressive medications also can alter the bacteria present in the body's ecosystem; these are typically prescribed or available over the counter to help reduce problems related to gastric acidity, such as acid reflux or ulcers, and commonly known versions of these "antacids" include histamine-2 blockers (ranitidine [Zantac])* and proton pump inhibitors (lansoprazole [Prevacid]). These drugs are not only among the most commonly used over-the-counter drugs taken by adults for heartburn, but they are often given to infants who regurgitate food and appear fussy. For the vast majority of infants, however, severe gastroesophageal reflux does not cause disease and it's a developmentally normal process. Adults also tend to overprescribe them to themselves because they are easy to obtain. They may be relieving one problem while igniting another.

According to Dr. Edward Mitre, an associate professor in the Department of Microbiology and Immunology at the Uniformed Services University in Bethesda, Maryland, 8 percent of all children in his team's study—nearly 800,000 infants—received a prescription for acid-suppressive therapy. The study's bold conclusions were compelling: "The hazard of developing an allergic disease was significantly increased in those who had received acid-suppressive medications or antibiotics during the first 6 months of life." They documented an increased risk of nearly every allergic disease they assessed (food allergy, anaphylaxis, asthma, atopic dermatitis, hay fever, allergic conjunctivitis, hives, contact dermatitis, medication allergy, and a class of other allergies). The only allergy they didn't show a link for was seafood allergy. The dosage of the medications also played a role in the association. Infants prescribed more than sixty days of proton pump inhibitors, for example, had a 52 percent greater risk of being diagnosed with food allergy in childhood than did those prescribed sixty days or less.

When the researchers looked at the impact antibiotics had on allergy development, they found that, regardless of dose, antibiotics prescribed during infancy were associated with a greater than twofold risk of asthma in childhood. They concluded that "Acid-suppressive medications and

---

*In 2020, the FDA removed Zantac and all ranitidine products from the market due to a contaminant found that increases risk of cancer. At this writing, it's not known whether the products will return to the market, but surely other acid-reducing drugs remain readily available in both prescription form and over-the-counter.

antibiotics should be used during infancy only in situations of clear clinical benefit."

It's important to bear in mind that these findings are showing associations—not cause-and-effect relationships. So, taking these drugs alone will not necessarily cause allergies, but they do add to the inputs that tip the scale in favor of developing them—at any age. Antacids targeted at adults have especially come under fire in new studies showing just how powerful they may be in fomenting allergic storms. In 2019, a large review of health records covering more than eight million Austrians revealed that those who used drugs to suppress stomach acid were almost *twice* as likely to need drugs to control allergy symptoms. The risk was especially prominent among older folks: people over age sixty who used these drugs were more than *five times* as likely to also need an allergy medication. One of the underlying connections here is straightforward: when you take acid-suppressing drugs, the food you eat is not completely broken down into small enough pieces, so intact allergens are sent to the intestine, where they can cause an allergic reaction and inflammation. That reaction alone will also impact the microbiome with further downstream effects.

More research is needed to understand all of these mechanisms, but the emerging science is forcing us to rethink how quickly we as physicians should recommend or prescribe these drugs. By the same token, anyone who suffers from chronic heartburn (more than sixty million Americans experience a bout of it at least once a month) may want to think twice about habitually using these medicines and seek other strategies with the help of their physician or even a dietitian. In many instances, chronic heartburn can be easily and swiftly resolved with a few tweaks to the diet.

Amazing to think we can do so much with our dietary choices. Partaking of food is the one experience we all share no matter where we live, what we do, how old we are, or what heritage we carry. All across our remarkably diverse planet, eating is one of the few activities that is universal. While food can be a source of pain and illness, it's also how we can heal and, ultimately, thrive as you find what works for you and learn to live fearlessly.

Fearless Facts

→ The American Academy of Pediatrics recommends a protocol to promote early introduction of allergenic foods for babies for allergy prevention (see Appendix A for details). Pregnant women are no longer told to avoid common allergenic foods unless they have allergies or intolerances. One of the most significant risk factors for developing food allergies is severe eczema in the baby, so it's important to discuss this with your pediatrician and consider allergy testing or an allergist visit when your child is around four months old.

→ Research shows that great ways to promote robust immune health include regular exercise, restorative sleep, reducing toxic stress, not smoking, limiting alcohol, and avoiding harmful infections via washing hands and masking when appropriate.

→ It's important to support the health and function of the microbiome, which also helps to bolster immunity. This is chiefly achieved through a healthy diet that includes sources of probiotics and avoids the unnecessary use of medications like antibiotics and antacids that can adversely affect the microbiome.

→ Remember, food is medicine!

nine

THRIVE IN YOUR DAILY WORLD

Cracking the Label Codes and
Building Confidence to Live Fearlessly

W HEN YOU WALK INTO A GROCERY STORE THERE IS AN ENDLESS ARRAY OF decisions to make. I've gathered a lot from my epidemiological research that tell a staggering story. An allergy or intolerance to one of the top nine food allergens affects the purchasing decisions of eighty-five million people in the US alone; 71 percent of these individuals read labels for every single food purchase even if they have previously bought the item; 55 percent spend a few minutes or more reading labels before they purchase a product, taking extra time to ensure their product will be safe for them and their family; 28 percent buy only products that have allergen-friendly labeling on the packaging. And 6 percent of food allergic households avoid an entire food category (e.g., bread, snacks, frozen food) specifically due to a food allergy that someone in the family has. Such a trend gives way to a roughly $19 billion opportunity for those who avoid entire packaged food categories or purchase allergen alternative products.

As you can likely guess, gluten and dairy dominate allergen alternatives and make up 97 percent of the market, in large part due to the associated health halo even among people who may not medically be allergic to wheat or have celiac disease or nonceliac gluten sensitivity. Small brands have cornered this market, but the big brands are also getting into the lucrative game. Labels for gluten-free products are relatively easy to spot because food manufacturers know they can attract people with their gluten-free claims. But for many other potentially problematic ingredients, labeling practices fall short.

Although advisory labels are helpful, the widespread use of precautionary allergen labeling like "may contain" or "manufactured in . . . ," which represents "allergen traces" on prepackaged foods, can be difficult for families and can lead to anxiety and stress around shopping for packaged foods that are staples in many people's diet. The other issue involves the unintended "side effects," if you will, of extensive use of this labeling that dilutes their value. When you see copious warning labels everywhere, it's natural to gradually perceive those labels as not so dangerous or useful anymore. It's like seeing red lights blinking all the time to the point they lose their effect; but notice one glaring red light on occasion and it takes on more meaning. In one of my own studies, up to 40 percent of individuals admitted that they ignore "may contain" statements. What value do those labels have if they are ignored?

I've done a lot of work on these types of precautionary allergen labels (PALs), which are intended to warn consumers of potential undeclared allergens—ones that accidentally get into the food. Unfortunately, studies by my team and others have shown that these labels cause much confusion. One in three consumers falsely believed that precautionary allergen statements are based on the amounts of allergen in the product. Not so. These labels are not regulated and there are no standards that food manufacturers rely on to determine the wording that they use. If a "may contain" label meant that the food might have a threshold, such as up to 100 milligrams of an allergen, then patients could work with their doctor to find out just how much of their allergen may be safe to consume and purchase foods accordingly. Allergists are studying the use of threshold testing in their practices that could give more assurance to consumers with food allergies when purchasing foods with PALs. Similar to PALs, restaurants may provide precautionary statements (e.g., "We cannot guarantee that . . ."), but these, too, tend to be vague and inconsistent (again, the Food Allergen Labeling and Consumer Protection Act [FALCPA] only applies to packaged FDA-regulated foods but labeling requirements do extend to retail and food-service establishments that package, label, and offer products for human consumption—see Chapter 5). Until we have that kind of precision, standardized language, and full transparency across the food supply board, people are left on their own without a clear sense of how risky ingesting a food is. What's one to do?

Here are the steps I teach people to take so they stay safe and informed:

Step 1: Understand how and where to find allergen information on a label. If your allergen is one of the top nine, then you know FALCPA requires by law that packaged foods list an allergen in plain English if it is an ingredient. Note: Sesame was only recently made part of this legal list at the federal level in the US. Sesame labeling has been mandated in Canada, the European Union, Australia, and of course Illinois. Our Illinois congressman and friend Jonathan Carroll, who understands the issues as he has a daughter with food allergies, passed this law in Illinois for all sesame-containing items to be labeled as such, using the data from our lab (and I encourage people to use our data to advocate for similar important policy initiatives).

> **Warning:** Not all cookies and sandwiches are created equal. Foods produced in a bakery or deli and "placed in a wrapper or container in response to a consumer's order" are not covered under federal labeling requirements. So, when you decide to buy a fresh cookie to follow your turkey sandwich for lunch at the market's deli and bakery, the container you receive packed by the

continues

continued

store worker will not have any federally regulated allergen labels on it even though the food inside may indeed contain problematic ingredients. For this reason, it's important to ask questions at the counter; and if food service workers are not able to give you clear answers about allergens and potential cross-contact with other items they are selling, speak with a supervisor or store manager. When in doubt, take it out (of your shopping cart).

Other exclusions to be aware of: FALCPA does not enforce labeling on prescription and over-the counter drugs, personal care items (e.g., cosmetics, shampoo, mouthwash, toothpaste, or shaving cream), pet foods and supplies, any food products regulated by the United States Department of Agriculture (USDA) Food Safety and Inspection Service (FSIS) (e.g., meat and poultry products and whole eggs), or any food product regulated by the Alcohol and Tobacco Tax and Trade Bureau. Although the USDA FSIS encourages food companies to follow FALCPA, they are not obligated to do so. What's more, highly refined oils from soybean and raw agricultural commodities, such as fresh fruits and vegetables, are also exempt from source labeling. Highly refined oils, however, are not usually problematic because the refining process substantially reduces the allergenicity of oils; it's the unrefined (cold-pressed, expelled, extruded) oil that are most likely to elicit a reaction. Raw agricultural products (e.g., corn, rice) may contain low levels of a different allergenic crop (e.g., soybean or wheat) due to shared farm equipment, and are infrequently labeled.

Read ingredient lists carefully and become familiar with the scientific names for your allergen so you are able to identify them in their various forms. Familiarize yourself with common hiding places for your allergen. The following is a chart adapted from one of my own papers that shows how pervasive many hidden food allergens can be in the food supply. For a more comprehensive list, go to www.foodwithoutfearbook.com.

Foods Containing Major Allergens and Alternative Names for Major Food Allergens

(Adapted from the FARE website on food avoidance.)

MAJOR ALLERGEN	FOOD ALLERGENS/FOODS CONTAINING ALLERGEN	ALTERNATIVE NAMES FOR ALLERGEN OR ALLERGEN COMPONENT
Milk	Milk (all forms of cow's, sheep's, and goat's milk), butter, buttermilk, cheese, condensed milk, cottage cheese, cream, cream cheese, curds, half-and-half, ice cream, milk powder, milk solids, nonfat milk solids, sherbet, sour cream, whipped cream, yogurt *May Contain Milk:* Artificial butter or "butter-flavored" products, baked goods, butter, candies, canned meats, cereal, chocolate, cookies, custard, deli meat, ghee, some medications, some pareve products; some pretzels and definitely cheese-flavored snacks, also some fried potato products	Casein, casein hydrolate, caseinates, curd, diacetyl, lactalbumin, lactoferrin, lactoglobulin, lactose, lactulose, recaldent, rennet casein, sodium caseinate, tagatose, whey, whey protein hydrolysate
Egg	Eggs (including turkey, quail, duck, and goose, as they are cross-reactive with chicken eggs), albumin, dried egg, eggnog, powdered egg, egg protein, egg white, egg yolk, globulin, nonvegan mayonnaise, meringue, surimi, tamago *May Contain Egg:* Baked goods, Caesar dressing, candy, cakes, cookies, French toast, fried foods, ice cream, marshmallows, nougat, pasta, pretzels, puddings/custards	Albumin, lysozyme, ovalbumin, ovomucin, ovomucoid, ovovitellin, lecithin (most lecithin in the US are based on soy and allowed for those with egg allergies), livetin, vitellin

continues

continued

MAJOR ALLERGEN	FOOD ALLERGENS/FOODS CONTAINING ALLERGEN	ALTERNATIVE NAMES FOR ALLERGEN OR ALLERGEN COMPONENT
Peanut	Peanuts, beer nuts, cold-pressed peanut oil, goobers/goober peas, ground nuts, mixed nuts, monkey nuts, nutmeat, nut pieces, peanut butter, peanut flour, peanut kernels, peanut oil, Valencias *May Contain Peanut:* African, Asian, and some Mexican foods, baked goods, BBQ sauce, candy, chocolate, chili/hot sauces, glazes/marinades, gravy, mole and enchilada sauce, nougat, piecrust, trail mixes	Arachide, arachis, arachis oil, peanut protein hydrolysate
Tree nuts	Almonds, beechnut, Brazil nut, butternut, cashew, chestnut, chinquapin, ginkgo nut, hazelnut/filbert, lychee nut, macadamia nut, marzipan, pecan/hickory nut, pesto, pine nut, pistachio, praline, walnut, nut extracts and alcoholic extracts (e.g., Amaretto), nut butters, nut meal, nutmeat, nut oils, nut paste, nut pieces	
Wheat	Bread crumbs, baked goods, bulgur, cereal extract, cereals, couscous, cracker meal, flour (all-purpose, bread, cake, durum, enriched, graham, gravies, pastry, self-rising, soft wheat, stone-ground, whole wheat, etc.), hydrolyzed wheat protein, kamut, matzo, matzo meal, pasta, seitan, semolina, spelt, sprouted wheat, wheat starch, whole wheat berries; also, soy sauce, surimi *May Contain Wheat:* Baked goods, bread crumbs, candies, caramel color, chocolates, crackers, gravies, hot dogs, ice cream, matzo, noodles, pasta, processed meats, pretzels, soy sauces, thicker soups	Durum, einkorn, emmer, farina, farro, triticale, sprouted wheat (bran, germ, gluten, grass, malt, starch), vital wheat gluten, wheat bran hydrolysate, wheat germ oil, wheatgrass, wheat protein isolate

MAJOR ALLERGEN	FOOD ALLERGENS/FOODS CONTAINING ALLERGEN	ALTERNATIVE NAMES FOR ALLERGEN OR ALLERGEN COMPONENT
Finfish	Anchovies, bass, catfish, caviar, cod, flounder, grouper, haddock, hake, herring, mahimahi, monkfish, orange roughy, perch, pike, pollack, salmon, sardines, scrod, sole, smelt, snapper, swordfish, tilapia, trout, tuna, whitefish, whiting, and other finfish *May Contain Fish:* Bonito broth, Caesar salad dressing, fish oil supplements, fish sauce, fish stock, gumbo, imitation crab, kosher gelatin or isinglass, paella, surimi, Worcestershire sauce	
Shellfish	Crustaceans: barnacle, crab, crawfish, krill, lobster (langouste, langoustine) scampi, prawns, shrimp Mollusks: abalone, clams, cockle, cuttlefish, mussels, octopus, oyster, oyster sauce, scallops Other: sea cucumber, sea urchin, snails (escargot), squid (calamari) *May Contain Shellfish:* Bouillabaisse, fish stock, paella, seafood flavoring, oyster sauce	
Soy	Soybeans (soya), edamame, hydrolyzed soy protein, miso, natto, shoyu, soy cheese, soy fiber, soy flour, soy grits, soy ice cream, soy milk, soy noodles, soy nuts, soy powder, soy protein, soy protein isolate, soy sauce, soy sprouts, soy yogurt, tamari, tempeh, textured soy protein (TSP), textured vegetable protein (TVP), tofu *May Contain Soy:* Cereals, energy bars, processed deli meats, vegetable broth, vegetable oils and shortenings, veggie burgers and sausage	

continues

continued

MAJOR ALLERGEN	FOOD ALLERGENS/FOODS CONTAINING ALLERGEN	ALTERNATIVE NAMES FOR ALLERGEN OR ALLERGEN COMPONENT
Sesame	Sesame seed, gomasio (sesame salt), sesame seed oil, tahina, tahini *May Contain Sesame:* Asian food, baked goods, bread crumbs, cereals, chips, crackers, dressing and dips, falafel, halvah, hummus, Middle Eastern foods and desserts, pasteli, snacks, soups, sushi	Benne seed (gingelly seed, sesamolina, sesamum indicum, sim sim, tehina, til) Other seeds that could be problematic: flax, hemp, poppy, sunflower

Spices and colorings can also contain allergens but, again, only the top eight are required to be listed. The only way to know if a product contains another suspected allergen is to call the manufacturer or check the manufacturer's website for more detailed information (look for allergen information or FAQs sections). While this can be time-consuming, it can give you the information you need and can then rely on for future decisions. Many of my patients find it helpful to avoid any products that have precautionary labels and seek foods that are made in allergen-free facilities. But other patients find this too limiting, in which case we work together to develop a plan that strikes an appropriate balance between risk vs. benefit.

The analogy we like to use in medicine is to think about the risk of crossing the street. Anyone can be at risk of an accident when crossing a road, but usually you can gauge the level of risk by how much traffic there is and how perilous it might be to cross at any given time, given walk signs, and traffic signals. In some instances, you may choose to not cross the road altogether and find another path (the equivalent of another food or restaurant). Note, too, that ingredients in products and/ or the manufacturing process can change at any time. The best defense is to read labels each and every time before consuming. Also bear in mind that someone allergic to cow's milk would likely react to milk from sheep, goats, and maybe camels. And someone allergic to chicken eggs would also likely react to eggs from other birds.

Step 2: Understand cross-contact and know where to find label warnings. Cross-contact is when a food allergen accidentally gets into food. (Note: sometimes you may hear someone call it cross-contamination, though that terminology is technically saved for the process by which bacteria or another microorganism are unintentionally transferred from one substance or object to another, with harmful effects, such as salmonella food poisoning.) Cross-contact usually happens in small amounts, perhaps even microscopic, and can be difficult to detect. One Canadian study found that 17 percent of accidental exposures were caused by foods that had no advisory label but contained allergen due to cross-contact during manufacturing or processing. Once again, here in the US, the federal government does not require manufacturers to include labeling for possible cross-contact of allergens, but some manufacturers take on the responsibility themselves and often use unregulated precautionary statements to warn consumers of potential risks in certain food products. As a reminder, examples include:

"May contain traces of X"

"Manufactured on equipment that uses or processes X"

"Processed in a facility that processes X, Y, and Z"

Other commonly used labels include "Made on shared equipment with X," and "Not guaranteed to be free of X." The unregulated nature of these labels can make for a confusing array of language employed across different brands and manufacturers, as meanings can differ from company to company. There is no indication that one precautionary statement is safer than another and putting trust in one over another is not advised. In our recent study on this topic, my team found that consumers decide, based on the wording of precautionary allergen labels, what seems safe for themselves or their child. My team and I are currently working on policies that will clarify the "May contain" label.

We're also working with national organizations to advocate for better threshold amounts in the foods that carry these labels.

Although preventing cross-contact even in a highly controlled home environment can be difficult, there are strategies that can be implemented to make things easier. Examples include: Washing hands and cooking utensils as well as chopping boards and work surfaces well when preparing food; cooking different foods in clean oil and well-washed pans and using separate serving spoons for each dish. In addition, use clean dish towels and cleaning rags to avoid spreading allergens. Eating outside of the home is the greater challenge, especially in places where accidental exposures due to cross-contact commonly occur (think: buffets, salad bars, ice-cream parlors, ethnic restaurants, and bakeries). If you're eating in a restaurant, it's up to you to speak to the server and preferably cook/chef to let them know about the allergy and to ask questions about ingredients in foods and possible cross-contact. In ice-cream parlors, for example, scoops should not be shared between different ice cream tubs but they often are.

Although a rare occurrence, sometimes the labels are just plain wrong. In 2018, about one-third of FDA recalls involved prepackaged foods that were erroneously labeled. In the summer of 2020, the FDA recalled pastries from Whole Foods Market that contained undeclared egg, as well as Key lime tartlets with undeclared almond. (To access a full list of FDA- and USDA-issued recalls, go to https://www.foodsafety.gov/recalls-and-outbreaks. Sign up for food allergy recalls: Accidents happen and thankfully the FDA and USDA release food allergy recalls and warnings for undeclared allergens. Sign up for their alerts to receive emails directly.)

Be on the Lookout, but Also Be Ready and Equipped

Even the most careful and conscientious of people may someday accidentally ingest an allergen that elicits a dangerous reaction. Unintentionally eating a piece of fruit that gives you oral allergy syndrome or downing a cake that contains an additive that upsets your stomach will have uncomfortable consequences that are largely tolerable (not to mention survivable!)—you'll get through the reaction and learn to avoid those foods in the future. But serious IgE-mediated reactions to a food allergen demand greater vigilance and attention because these, as you know, are the reactions that can be severe and life-threatening.

Anyone with an IgE-mediated allergy should have emergency medications to treat reactions on hand at all times. This means having a prescribed epinephrine autoinjector, ideally two, in case multiple doses are needed, or there's a misfire on the first attempt as happened with Susan. Intramuscular epinephrine (injected in the middle of the outer side of the thigh) is the first line of treatment for all cases of anaphylaxis. The general rule is that epinephrine should be given to patients experiencing systemic symptoms involving the respiratory and/or cardiovascular system Sever symptoms involving two organ systems, such as the skin (multiple hives) and gastrointestinal tract, or rapidly progressive reaction (profuse vomiting or widespread hives) should also be treated with epinephrine. Of course, all patients who receive these prescriptions should be instructed on how to use the autoinjector correctly.

I have personally experienced and heard from so many how difficult it is to make a clear assessment in the heat of the moment. I want to be very clear that if ever in doubt, do not hesitate to use epinephrine. It is a very safe medication. Other drugs could also be prescribed to have at the ready as well to address certain symptoms, such as antihistamines ("H1 blockers," such as Benadryl) for skin symptoms, and short-acting bronchodilators, such as albuterol, for people with asthma. Again, the needs of each individual patient must be addressed. If respiratory symptoms are occurring, epinephrine should be given first and then the inhaler. Additional medications that may be given in the emergency room include oxygen, corticosteroids, H2 blockers, pressors, and intravenous fluids.

EPI SMARTS

+ Recognize the severity and act quickly.
+ Use epinephrine immediately.
+ Call 911.
+ Carry two autoinjectors.
+ Follow up. Discuss with your primary care doctor and allergist annually.

TRAVEL SMARTS

Individuals and families in the early stages of dealing with food allergy often limit traveling—notably via airplane or to unfamiliar foreign countries—for fear they won't be in control of encounters with food allergens. Regardless of age and experience with food allergy, travel can be extra daunting if you're going to countries where cultural and language barriers pose added challenges. When traveling on airplanes it is advisable to check out the airline's policies about food allergies and see whether you can alert them about any special circumstances you may have. For example, some airlines may allow individuals to preboard and wipe down the seating area and table. This is helpful especially if the allergic individual is a young child. It is also reasonable to carry your own food for the flight and bring all prescription medications on board including auto-injectable epinephrine, antihistamines, and asthma inhalers. If you're traveling alone, wearing medical alert jewelry can add another layer of protection.

In an international survey of people with peanut and tree nut allergies led by a group at the University of Michigan, it was found that 349 of 3,273 participants had a reaction in flight and 13.3 percent received epinephrine as treatment. The study suggested that requesting certain accommodations during air travel might lower the odds of having a reaction. You can, for example, ask that the airline announce to passengers that they avoid eating peanut-/tree nut–containing goods, and avoid the airline-provided pillows and blankets. Also, take your own wipes and clean the area around where you will be sitting. I have had a few occasions when the flight I was on requested a doctor for an ill passenger. Over the years, I have looked into the in-flight emergency medical kit and found epinephrine autoinjectors. I was very impressed and happy to see that this is now included on many airline flight kits.

It's a good idea to learn the words for your food allergen in the language of your destination. It is recommended to have a written statement (such as a chef card; see below) to show to hotel and restaurant staff stating what the allergen is and that eating it can cause a severe reaction. My family took a chef card in Italian to Italy and showed it when we dined. My daughter Riya was very nervous the first time, but when the chef read it out loud and fully understood it in front of her, he promised to make something amazing. That meal was the best pasta she has ever had and she felt so special and cared for.

THE CHEF CARD

Carrying a chef card can be a good idea for families that like to eat out and worry about encountering problematic foods. These cards outline the foods one must avoid and can be the ideal way to communicate food allergies to a chef or manager at restaurants. The FARE website provides an interactive PDF of chef card templates in English and a number of foreign languages to use while traveling or at ethnic food restaurants: www.foodallergy.org/life-food-allergies/managing-lifes-milestones/dining-out/food-allergy-chef-cards.

DIGITAL SMARTS

As we increasingly shift to electronic medical records, and those records are shared among different health-care centers, it's important to ensure your allergens and other problematic foods or ingredients be properly recorded. If and when you land in a hospital and your doctors access your profile in making important decisions about your care and treatment, you'll want the information to be accurate—and comprehensive. You may not be in a position to articulate your allergies and sensitivities, or you might assume that your health record speaks for itself.

You likely have written your allergies down on a questionnaire at some point in your doctor's office or in an ER and assumed it was all entered correctly and comprehensively into the system. But that may not have been the case. Now that most patients have access to a patient portal online, it's vital to check that your data and all allergies and sensitivities are correctly noted. This is especially important if you are in a situation where you're not under your usual physician's care or happen to be in a hospital or medical setting outside of your typical setting or network. Your smartphone probably has as digital medical ID that can help store information as well. Get to know these technologies and use them wherever possible.

MINDING THE MIND

Food is not only essential to our body, it is also often a core component of social and religious life. Therefore, it is no surprise that adverse reactions to food can not only be physically unpleasant, but also emotionally devastating. A child who can no longer eat their favorite foods like cake and cookies, out of fear of an allergic reaction, an adult who can no longer grab food from a shared plate without thinking twice about possibly hidden ingredients or cross-contact—these are but a few of the ways that food-related conditions can impact one's psychological and social well-being. Overly restricted diets can even compromise balanced nutrition and reduce energy levels. This contributes to a cycle of negative experiences and potentially negative self-appraisals and mood.

Life following the first adverse reaction to a food is often accompanied by growing uncertainty and even anxiety. Anxiety grows because of that uncertainty and discomfort. The classic "what if" questions are tell-tale indicators of anxious thinking. That is, one is worrying about something that hasn't happened yet.

Am I allergic to other foods now? What will happen if I am accidentally exposed again? Could my next reaction be life-threatening? Am I going to have to worry about this for the rest of my life? These are only a few of the many concerns that my patients have shared with me after their initial adverse reaction to a food. For parents of children with suspected food allergy, their concern can be even greater than those related by the patients themselves.

Any health diagnosis can be overwhelming and psychologically troubling, especially when there's no guaranteed cure and you learn that it's a chronic condition in need of ongoing management. Additionally, food allergies are unique in that they are asymptomatic until there is an allergic reaction. Consequently, it's really an invisible or hidden chronic illness. It's totally normal for food allergy patients and their families to experience anxiety and emotional distress as a result of their food allergies. But as a physician and advocate for food allergy patients, I think it's important to provide useful information, tools, and tips to cope with the challenges of living with a food allergy.

While it's true that some studies have found rates of anxiety and other adverse mental health outcomes to be more common among food allergy patients and their families, compared to their nonallergic counterparts, it is important to remember that with support and resources patients and families are able to successfully manage their food allergies along with the anxiety and stress that go with it. Furthermore, we have learned so much about food-related conditions in the past few years, how to treat them, and how to effectively support patients that we are entering a new era—one where food-related conditions are another one of life's many challenges that can be surmounted with the help of modern medicine and an effective support network. When counseling my patients, I often find it helpful to apply the "Goldilocks Principle," which can be understood using the diagram below.

According to this "Goldilocks" principle, there exists an optimal level of anxiety that helps patients/caregivers to effectively cope and manage their allergy while at the same time reducing the likelihood that patients/caregivers engage in unnecessary fear-driven hypervigilance or potentially dangerous risk-taking behavior. Since it's impossible to reduce risk to 0 percent, I try to encourage my patients to achieve an attitude of "relaxed readiness" where they are prepared to identify and treat an accidental reaction, but do not allow their fear and anxiety to overwhelm them. "Relaxed readiness" highlights the integration of several coping strategies. It combines accurate information gathering (a cognitive coping strategy), feeling regulation (an emotional or self-regulation coping strategy), and practice (a behavioral experience that helps patterns become automatic responses).

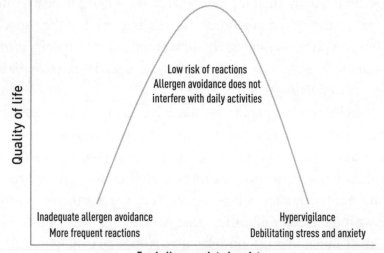

To achieve a healthier, more balanced attitude about food-related conditions, and how to best manage them, it is essential to consult an expert. For patients with a suspected food allergy, this almost always involves a consultation with a board-certified allergist. It is also important to consult a psychologist trained in food allergy, and a dietitian as needed. My research suggests that there are millions of Americans who incorrectly believe themselves to be food allergic, and therefore are likely avoiding foods unnecessarily and adversely impacting their quality of life in the process. In extreme cases, such avoidance can spiral into an eating disorder. Therapists who counsel people with eating disorders will tell you that they see a lot of individuals whose disordered, unhealthy relationship with food owe at least some of their origins to food allergies and intolerances.

Granted, I should temper this by saying that such cases are rare, but there's a gradual awareness among health practitioners about the link between any condition on the food allergy spectrum and eating disorders. After all, the two share a common behavioral reality: preoccupation with—fear of—food. And they both share a feeling of being imprisoned by food and decisions around food, for which freedom comes with learning how to have a healthy relationship with it and make smart, health-promoting choices based on individual needs, preferences, and any underlying conditions. These are some warning signs that quality of life has declined and is interfering with optimal functioning: preoccupied thinking, organizing all of your behaviors around food avoidance, anxiety that spills into other areas of life and then derails typical social and emotional functioning in school and/or work, sleep problems, irritability that interferes with significant relationships, and so forth. Behavioral health interventions including mindfulness practices and guided imagery, journaling, virtual and in-person support groups, individual therapy, and family consultation can help change these problem thoughts, feelings, and behaviors.

I didn't use the term "food freedom" randomly in this book. It's a term with many meanings. Imagine the relief of finding out that you're not actually allergic to dairy and wheat, after years of avoiding these delicious staples! Sometimes all it takes is a single visit to an allergist office where the suspected allergen can be consumed under strict supervision (e.g., an oral food challenge). Remarkably, studies show that patient and caregiver quality of life can improve substantially after participating in an oral food challenge—no matter whether the challenge rules out the allergy or confirms it! In this case, knowledge really is power. This beautifully illustrates how anxiety "feeds" off of uncertainty, and when the level of uncertainty is reduced (regardless of whether it confirms or disconfirms a food allergy), one's experience is improved.

Sometimes obtaining this knowledge can be uncomfortable, but worth it in the long run. For example, much of the fear is due to the deaths we hear about from food allergic reactions. The fact is suffering a fatal outcome from food allergy is incredibly rare. A recent study by my colleague Dr. Paul Turner again spoke to the chances of a US patient dying from a food allergy being substantially low (less than 1 in 10 million). Many of the families that have suffered the loss of their children from these fatal reactions have started foundations to help educate the community about how to recognize a reaction and what to do, including how to use epinephrine. These foundations also encourage you to get a proper food allergy diagnosis and management tools from an allergist.

I have long believed in the power of a positive mind-set to reduce stress and improve health. Thankfully, recent studies have begun to provide compelling evidence in support of this as well. One notable study, carried out by my colleagues at Stanford, tested whether food allergy patients who were receiving oral immunotherapy might have a better outcome if they were primed to perceive any non-life-threatening allergy symptoms they experienced during treatment as "positive signals" that the treatment is working—instead of the traditional interpretation that they are "unfortunate side effects of treatment." This is important since many patients discontinue immunotherapy due to safety concerns after experiencing treatment-related symptoms (e.g., itchy mouth, congestion), when in fact these symptoms are not usually dangerous. They are simply par for the course.

Remarkably, people randomized to receive counseling that "symptoms are positive signals" experienced reduced anxiety and fewer symptoms, viewed their treatment more favorably, and had a better outcome compared to those randomized to treatment as usual (where any side effects were perceived as unfortunate side effects of treatment). I think this study is a great example of how small changes in how we physicians care for our patients can make a very big difference. It also highlights the key role that counseling and mental health care can play in helping food allergy patients and their families improve their quality of life. The more they know and understand what they are going through and what to expect, the better they can manage, see themselves through their treatment, and find some semblance of success. Our team, led by clinical psychologist Lisa Lombard, is now working on developing a virtual reality tool to help patients visualize treatment in a positive way and reduce their anxiety prior to and potentially during treatment.

Many families find counseling and support groups where they can share their experience and gain insights and encouragement from others to be incredibly valuable. As they say, it takes a village to raise a child, but it also takes a village to live with food allergy and build resiliency every step of the way regardless of age. Just ask Fritzie Shinohara, who went from fearsome to fearless in her mission to keep her family safe.

Like so many military families, Fritzie and her US Air Force husband found themselves moving a lot—Georgia, Virginia, Colorado, Illinois, and then back to Virginia. Fritzie was a civilian in the US Navy, working as a pharmacist before devoting all of her time to allergy advocacy work; they had to move every two years, which made it exceptionally difficult to manage their children's food allergies. Their three girls all had multiple food allergies, and with every move came new doctors and new schools, as well as financial hardships from shouldering the weight of managing their daughters' food allergies on a military income. Right before I met them in 2016, their eldest daughter, then aged eight, had lost her hair, a rare condition called alopecia totalis, whose cause is unknown but it's thought to be autoimmune. She'd gone through cycles of hair loss since the second grade, and also suffered from EoE. Grappling with drastic hair loss alone is enough to send an individual's mental state downhill, but add the extra challenge of multiple food allergies, and you can appreciate the warrior-like stance Fritzie and her husband had to take.

Fortunately, the family received a scholarship to attend our conference on food allergy, one that I and my team developed to support children and their families become more empowered dealing with their food allergies. This is where I met this wonderful family. Today, if you ask Fritzie what her lifeline was, she'll tell you that there's nothing more valuable to a parent of a child with food allergy than talking to other parents. "The number one thing to do is establish a support system in your community; find a local food allergy support group and attend a conference if you can," she says. "Get educated no matter how you go about that. Be your own advocate."

Great advice. I'll add that you don't have to be a parent of an allergic child to do these things. Anyone with a food-related condition would do well to seek a support group. They are cropping up everywhere now both in person and online. We have a list in Appendix B of many organizations and support groups. In fact, Fritzie has created her own Facebook group and founded a support group exclusive to military families. She's all about being your own advocate and taking control. And she's achieved just that. Fritzie no longer wonders why or how her daughters developed food allergy—she simply forges on with knowledge and confidence that will see her daughters through to become thoughtful, independent, and productive adults.

Fearless Facts

→ Part of learning how to live—and thrive—no matter where you are on the spectrum is knowing how to read labels and identify problematic ingredients, including those that can result from cross-contact. Precautionary allergen labels (PALs) serve a purpose and are helpful, but they often fall short of full transparency because they are not as tightly regulated or universally used across all potential substances that can cause reactions as people think. Many exclusions apply.

→ Common allergens (e.g., milk) can be listed under different names (e.g., casein) on food labels. It helps to be label literate and have the knowledge to easily interpret lists of ingredients without wholly relying on vague precautionary statements. To reduce risk of accidental allergen exposure, you may want to avoid any products that have precautionary labels and seek foods that are made in allergen-free facilities.

→ For people with bona fide food allergies that can lead to anaphylaxis, it's vital to be "epi smart" and know how to carry and use epinephrine when necessary. Ideally, carry two auto-injectors and do not hesitate to use them; it's a safe medicine.

→ For peace of mind and ease while traveling, carrying a chef card (see page 235) adds another layer of protection beyond your own vigilance and can help you to safely communicate your allergy and effectively navigate foreign culinary adventures.

→ Do not assume your medical records on file contain an accurate list of all of your allergies and sensitivities. These records are dynamic and it's important to make sure they are up to date and comprehensive. Don't be shy about informing others about your food-related condition, especially your clinical care providers.

→ Managing a chronic condition can be psychologically burdensome. To achieve true food freedom, you have to mend the mind as much as the body. Seek support from friends, family, and groups designed to address the same issues you're going through.

ACT LOCALLY, THINK GLOBALLY

What We Can Do as a Society to Turn This Epidemic Around

E VERY SINGLE PERSON WHO READS THIS BOOK HAS SOMETHING IN COMMON besides food issues. We all have gone through one of the most historic events in our lifetime with the novel coronavirus pandemic that began in 2020. Practically overnight, each one of us had to change how we worked, shopped, dined out, dressed, socialized, connected, traveled, vacationed, celebrated, parented, played, voted, enjoyed such entertainment as concerts and sports, and lived life in general. Nobody has been untouched by the virus's swift spread around the world, even if they've escaped infection. It has taught us a lot about ourselves, our environment, and the planet's delicate balance.

Although scientists have rightfully predicted such a pandemic for decades not knowing exactly when it would eventually strike, it still came as a surprise for many of us; perhaps we'd been in denial and diverted our attention to prepare for other threats, such as terrorist attacks and cybersecurity breaches. It can be hard for us humans to prepare for something that neither we nor our parents have experienced before and that may not take place in our own generation. We readily take the necessary steps to mitigate natural disasters and seasonal incidents, such as hurricanes and blizzards, because they happen with frequency and predictability. But a public health crisis on the scale of Covid-19? If you had been forewarned in 2010 of what could unfold a decade later, you might have been skeptical; a once-in-a-century pathogen and resulting pandemic that decimates society and its economies seem so remote in the mind as to be inconceivable.

The chances of a pandemic happening are the same tomorrow as they were yesterday and remain today, but no doubt our perceptions have changed immensely. We will live increasingly with the threat of a bug, probably of viral origin, taking shape in human-to-human transmission and wreaking global havoc. The confluence of climate change, deforestation, habitat loss, human migration, mass rapid transit, and aggressive conversion of wildland for economic development paves the way for making outbreaks of disease more common and more dangerous.

Aaron Bernstein is the interim director for the C-Change Center for Climate, Health, and the Global Environment at Harvard University's T. H. Chan School of Public Health. He is also a hospitalist in the Division of General Pediatrics at Boston Children's Hospital and specializes in studying how diseases emerge in a changing environment, notably the relationship between climate change and infectious disease. In a 2020 interview he did for ProPublica on Covid-19, he stated it bluntly: the idea that climate and health and environmental policy might not be related is "a dangerous delusion."

This statement reflects a similar sentiment shared by my colleagues in food allergy. Although not an infectious disease, food allergy (and all its iterations) is a major public health concern. Virtually every peer-reviewed paper on food allergy clearly states this, but if you were to ask anyone in the general public if they knew this fact, you'd find that most people have no clue—just as most people had no clue an infectious pandemic of epic proportions could happen. And contrary to conventional wisdom, the rise in food-related conditions owes its origins to some of the same circumstances that set the stage for viral pandemics. In a world where our environment is quickly changing, faster than our genome, it's no wonder we find our body rebelling against previously innocuous ingredients. Respecting the deep connections among climate, health, and environmental policies will not only help us prevent future pandemics, but it will also help us end food allergy. Technology will also serve a big role.

Picture a day when you can carry an app on your smartphone that can scan foods for potential allergens. Mobile apps already exist that, at the tap of a button on a home screen, can help you find allergen-friendly establishments (see Appendix B) or alert first responders and designated emergency contacts about an anaphylactic situation. Or how about hypoallergenic tree nuts and peanuts that have been genetically modified to be free of those troublsome proteins. Similarly, think of gene therapy that can safely edit your genome so your body never mistakes a certain food—or food group—for being villainous. All of these possibilities will likely be part of our future and some are already in development. In fact, portable devices that are like test tubes in your pocket, able to sense gluten or peanut in your food, are already beginning to emerge on the market (though most of these products need more advanced technology at less cost to be truly accessible to everyone). Food allergy vaccines likely will also be in our future, as more than a dozen pharmaceutical companies now have research and development programs focused on food allergy. The goal is to enhance the body's immune response by making the peanut allergen resemble an invading virus. Unlike oral immunotherapy that retrains the immune system to recognize allergens as harmless (in essence, disarming the immune system to some degree), the premise of a food vaccine is the opposite—to induce protective antibodies in a way more akin to traditional vaccination (in essence, arming the immune system so that it is prepared to identify and tolerate potentially allergenic proteins—such as peanut—immediately upon subsequent exposure).

I envision more options in the next few years, from vaccines to biologics to immunotherapy, with predictive modeling to see which one will work best for an individual taking into account genetics, microbiome, and a host of other factors. Additionally, as discussed earlier, many improved diagnostics are in the works, which we anticipate will usher in a future where adverse food reactions will not only be more quickly and reliably diagnosed, but that the resulting diagnosis can also include an indication of the anticipated severity of disease. Currently disease severity is largely reliant on classification of adverse reactions *after* they occur, but the next generation of diagnostic approaches aspires to provide patients and doctors with an estimate of a patient's risk of experiencing a severe reaction *before* it happens. This could be a true game changer. The volume of research that's happening now as you read this is astonishing. Compared to when I started in the field seventeen years ago, so many researchers and industry partners are getting involved and finding answers. And there's lots to gain on many levels beyond just improving the quality of life of millions of sufferers. Analysts predict that the food allergy treatment market will reach $40 billion by 2025.

These innovations are not fantasy. In fact, each of the aforementioned technologies are currently in different phases of development and I suspect many will become commonplace in the coming years, serving as a complement to the various food allergy treatments described in Chapter 7. I expect advancements to happen in the realm of addressing food intolerances as well, an area that begs to be more science-driven and effective. A revolution is under way in my field and I'm both excited and optimistic about the future. When my career shifted into food allergy research more than a decade ago, the National Institutes of Health barely funded the field; now it's considered a priority area.

At the same time, however, we need to be sure that these advances in food allergy management, treatment, and prevention remain within the grasp of every patient regardless of their financial means and access to health care. You'll recall Emily Brown from Chapter 6 who is founder and CEO of Kansas City's Food Equality Initiative, where she's placed over $100,000 worth of "free-from" food into the hands of her clients in need. A dedicated advocate for individuals facing food insecurity and managing a medically necessary diet, Emily passionately shares her personal experience with food insecurity and food allergies at speaking engagements with local nonprofits, health organizations, government leaders, and more.

Years ago, when she sought help from the Women, Infant & Children (WIC) program to help feed her own child, she soon learned that her daughter was unable to eat many of the foods offered by WIC due to her extensive allergies (peanut, milk, egg, wheat, and soy—the staples in so many foods). Emily then looked for assistance at local food pantries, but again, her daughter's allergies prevented her from taking full advantage of the foods the pantries offered. That experience ignited a fire within Emily to lead the charge in doing what she could to improve health and end hunger among individuals diagnosed with food allergies.

A food allergy diagnosis should not become a financial hardship, let alone one that's also emotional and physical. Much in the way that Covid-19 has unveiled health disparities across the nation, such inequities have plagued many other conditions for far too long, food allergy included. Everyone has to eat, but when it costs a family thousands of dollars more a year just to put nutritious food on the table that won't send a loved one to the ER, that fact alone plainly divides the haves and have-nots. Price is not the only barrier. It's also about access to the right food. "It's like peeling an onion," Emily remarks on the multilayered problem she tackles every day one step at a time. "In my work, I find that I peel one layer back and find another."

She also points to the food deserts out there, where people in rural areas and inner cities cannot find foods on local store shelves that will work with their dietary needs. She hopes that one day her daughter can try oral immunotherapy (OIT), which often entails out-of-pocket costs not covered by insurance in addition to the logistical complications that also increase expenses, commitments, and responsibilities. The frequent visits to the clinic performing the OIT, for example, has driven individuals and families to consider cross-country moves and job changes to accommodate and prioritize access to state-of-the-art food allergy treatment.

Our health-care system in its access, delivery, and insurance coverage is bound for renovations in the coming years. If there's a silver lining in the Covid-19 pandemic, it may very well be a welcomed hastening of health-care reform that will affect every patient no matter what ails them. On October 30, 2013, the CDC published the first national comprehensive guidelines for school food allergy management, "Voluntary Guidelines for Managing Food Allergies in Schools and Early Care and Education Programs." Although "voluntary," the guidelines are intended to support the implementation of school food allergy management policies in schools and early childhood programs, and guide improvements to existing practices.

Food allergy awareness has gained tremendous traction since I entered the field. I'm proud that the public school system in Chicago, where I live, was one of the first in the nation to implement policies mandating stocking epinephrine for emergency treatment of anaphylaxis. Unfortunately, this all was sparked by a young child dying at school after an anaphylactic reaction and there was no epinephrine. After that, the school system pledged not to let that ever happen again, passing a law to make epinephrine available in every public school in Chicago. Many of these deaths are preventable. Even close calls are preventable. Every time someone experiences a serious reaction, it can throw a person—and often their entire family—off course. It's hard to then go out to eat and do normal things, so avoiding those reactions entirely is important; and the good news is, we know how to do that via educational initiatives and awareness-raising. To see policies developed—to witness the community coming together to protect kids and adults with food allergy so quickly—is inspiring and should be an example for all citizens across the nation.

Statewide guidelines for school food allergy management have been published in a number of states, but my hope is that every state implements these guidelines. Multiple states also have passed legislation that permits, *but does not require*, various public venues to stock undesignated epinephrine for emergency use. Undesignated epinephrine means it has not been prescribed to any particular individual and is meant to be used on anyone in need of the drug (i.e., anyone experiencing anaphylaxis). This is the same concept as keeping defibrillators in public venues to facilitate prompt treatment of anyone experiencing cardiac arrest. Examples of public venues where undesignated epinephrine can be beneficial include day camps, youth recreation programs, theme parks, daycare centers, restaurants, sports arenas, and college campuses. A small number of states have passed laws specific to colleges and universities that allow, but do not require, these institutions to stock undesignated epinephrine. The laws differ by state, but may provide exemption from civil liability and outline specific requirements for training personnel, as well as how to maintain, store, and administer the epinephrine.

These public safety nets are built through the coordinated efforts of dedicated people affected by food allergy. As I have been in the food allergy field since 2004, I have seen the growth of many organizations and advocacy groups. I have had the privilege and honor to work with so many of them focusing on specific areas in food allergies, related conditions, such as asthma, eczema, EoE, and many others. I have attended and spoken at many of their meetings for families, physicians, researchers, educators, policymakers, and more. It is really so wonderful to see these organizations all coming together to discuss important issues that impact the community and to be a part of the conversation catalyzing change. You may be involved or aware of some that have been around for a long time, such as Allergy and Asthma Network (AAN), Asthma and Allergy Foundation of America (AAFA), FARE, and Food Allergy and Anaphylaxis Connection Team (FAACT), or newer ones like Food Allergy Fund and Allergy Strong. Many family foundations have joined the calling and new ones are developing every month.

You may feel powerless in the fight to change food allergy on a public health level or start an organization as Emily Brown did. But there's a lot you can do to help facilitate this revolution and play your part in ushering in real, positive change. Don't know where to start? Check out our longer list of organizations (and their websites) and support groups in Appendix B and get involved. There are many local and national groups that focus on policy, advocacy, peer support, education, and even clinical trials.

When Lisa Gable was named CEO of FARE in 2018, I knew we were in great hands to accelerate our mission in both public awareness about food allergy and research to inform new diagnostics and treatments. A former US ambassador, Gable has a reputation of being unrelentingly tenacious. "I knock the boulders out of the way," she says. "My goal is to bring together political parties, government agencies, corporations, research institutions, and individuals to create sustainable partnerships and programs that advance food allergy issues," pursuing "innovation as defined by usability."

FARE and its partner organizations understand that technology is only as good as its ability to be accessible. So, when we start to think about changes in how we identify and empower patients and their food-related conditions, push for more universal labeling, and democratize treatments and medicine, including novel therapies, such as OIT, which unfortunately remains unrealistic and impractical for many, such an approach is refreshing and, ultimately, effective. We must find affordable solutions for families across the board—and across the spectrum. FARE is a nonprofit but, under Gable's leadership, the organization has profoundly elevated funding and shined a light on the food allergy world as never before.

Another longtime advocate and friend I have known for over a decade is the president and CEO of the Allergy and Asthma Network, Tonya Winders. She is also the mother of five children, four of whom have asthma and/or allergies. Her hope and vision include "a day when we better understand the science in order to diagnose, treat, and potentially cure food allergies," recognizing the "significant strides in awareness and public policy over the past ten years."

No one understands food allergies better than those living with them every day. The stories and data collected by these organizations from your participation can help us researchers broaden our understanding and answer questions that will lead to important breakthroughs.

While I work closely with these organizations, my primary responsibility beyond my patients is as director of the Center for Food Allergy & Asthma Research (CFAAR) at Northwestern University Feinberg School of Medicine and Ann & Robert H. Lurie Children's Hospital of Chicago, where I and my team work to engage food allergy and asthma stakeholders in our local community in addition to our clinical commitments and research to better understand the physical, psychosocial, and economic burden of food allergy and asthma. We help build awareness and train the next generation through our summer internship program and training opportunities found on our website. Our center's research also studies how to optimize food allergy and asthma management, reduce disparities in care, implement school-based interventions, and advance policies to improve the lives of patients. We work very closely with the local school district—including Chicago Public Schools—and have developed videos (from daycare to college) that are free on our website and for schools to use addressing how to teach a classroom about food allergies and how to cultivate support among peers. Stomping out misinformation and bullying toward those with allergies starts with education. The site—www.feinberg.northwestern.edu/sites/cfaar/—is filled with useful resources and I encourage you to check it out.

Our team is currently working to reduce disparities and better understand differences in food allergy presentation, management, and access by race and socioeconomic status. After our earlier epidemiological work outlined the disparities in food allergy (mentioned on page 125), we developed the Food Allergy Management in Low Income Youth (FAMILY) study to begin identifying the mechanisms behind them. Using this data, we created the Food Allergy Passport and Workbook to try and mitigate some of them (free to download on our website). We are currently conducting the Food Allergy Outcomes Related to White and African American Racial Differences (FORWARD) study that follows Black, white, and Latinx families to identify differences in the disease and its burden. This is a collaborative with the National Institutes of Health (NIH) and our partner sites in Cincinnati (Cincinnati Children's Hospital led by Dr. Amal Assa'ad), Washington DC (DC Children's National led by Dr. Hemant Sharma), and Chicago (Rush University Medical Center led by Dr. Mary Tobin and our site at Lurie Children's Hospital).

As researchers, we have a profound potential to change our world. You might be familiar with the mantra "with evidence, change is possible" (from the organization Physicians for Human Rights). In this spirit, we work closely with multiple organizations to ensure our center's research synergizes with, and can fuel, their advocacy efforts. I encourage you to join us and get involved. We love the voice of the community and are passionate about learning from and participating in improving the health and lives of adults and children every day. We have developed a community advisory board that helps us come up with important topic areas for education and research and ensure that our work systematically addresses the most pressing concerns within our community.

I have a little cartoon on my wall at work and it embodies what I envision. It's an adult talking to a kid and the adult is saying, "You know, in my day there were no food allergies," because this is what you hear all the time today. Then, that kid grows up and has his chance to talk to a kid and says, "You know, in my day there were food allergies." Hopefully, that's where we're headed and it's thrilling to help be a part of that. Like Tonya and much of our community, I look forward to what the next decade will bring for my children and future grandchildren. My daughter, who is now a teenager, is still working through her peanut and tree nut allergy but has outgrown her egg allergy. She might always live with a nut allergy, but I have faith that she will enjoy life as an adult fearlessly.

Go to www.feinberg.northwestern.edu/sites/cfaar/ to stay up to date on our latest research, news, and upcoming events. There, you can also find a growing library of resources and help shape policies surrounding pediatric and adult allergic disease.

BE THE BUTTERFLY

It's often said that a butterfly flapping its wings can cause a tornado thousands of miles away. The so-called butterfly effect is a concept in chaos theory that suggests, put simply, that small events can have big effects. Credits go to the late Edward Norton Lorenz, a mathematician and meteorologist, who created the analogy in the late 1960s while he was establishing the theoretical basis of weather and climate predictability at MIT.

My point being: Be the butterfly. Do what you can in your family unit and community locally to effect massive global change. It's easier than you think.

Twenty years ago, you probably didn't know anyone who suffered from life-threatening allergies or who adhered to a gluten-free diet. Sure, you knew someone who couldn't eat anything with "traces of nuts," but hardly anybody carried an autoinjector syringe of epinephrine with them or avoided shrimp and lobster. Wheat-free diets were unheard of. FODMAP intolerance? Never. Compare that with this scenario as a reminder: Today at least 1 in 10 Americans is affected by food allergies, and at least 1 in 5 has an intolerance of some sort. For people with IgE-mediated allergies, you can't answer the question of "How severe is it?" There's no such thing as "mild" or "severe" because anyone can have an unwelcome reaction at the next bite that has never happened previously. And for people with intolerances, which could be confined to the gastrointestinal system, you can't label an intolerance as "moderate" in comparison, because the hit to their quality of life can also be devastating. Every point on the spectrum is troublesome.

Ending food allergies, intolerances, and masqueraders of all kinds will require a multipronged appreciation for the many, often-nuanced, contributing factors that come into play. The future of allergy control and eradicating food intolerances will not be through avoidance of certain foods and drug therapy alone. There has to be a better way. Those strategies will always be in the mix, but we must begin to look at the problem from a macro view. The road to an allergy-free future will rely heavily on prevention. As with so many conditions in medicine, it's usually much easier to prevent an ailment than to treat it, let alone cure it. Prevention in this realm will require attention to and possibly a shift in our lifestyle, and establishment of healthy habits that promote immune health.

Fight for Better Food Policy

As described earlier, the global food market is colossal. We have access to just about every kind of food year-round, with high-tech production of foods once found only in certain corners of the world or under certain seasonal conditions. And then there's the proliferation of new technologies sometimes used to make a food hardier, and other times used to create an entirely new food product. How do we develop better policies to safeguard our food supplies and bolster allergen management?

Part of my work entails reviewing food allergy policies so as to issue evidence-based recommendations for improving food safety for all. Much of this work is funded by the National Institutes of Health and will help communities, school systems, and public work environments adopt lifesaving policies. This is an important endeavor that will continue and increasingly recruit the wisdom of other researchers in various fields. As noted, we must galvanize the combined intelligence of experts in many different areas due to the prismatic complexities of food-related conditions. Just as there will not be a one-size-fits-all solution, neither is there a single path to the problem.

What you can do: Get engaged locally. Know where your local politicians stand on issues affecting your food environment and speak with them about measures that might make a difference. Start by simply writing to local politicians to lobby for changes that will help your neighborhood, your workplace, and beyond. Request changes at school, too, such as fewer meat-centric lunches, more time outside, and fewer harsh cleaning chemicals. If you live in or near a food desert where there is little access to fresh food, consider participating in Community Supported Agriculture (CSA) and community gardens (check out https://www.localharvest .org/csa/).

The Future of Medicine Is Inclusive

Allergies and food intolerances should not be siloed into a single area of discussion in scientific and wellness circles. As you've learned, the food reaction spectrum is wide and deep with a multitude of avenues where any single condition can involve multiple systems in the body. Such a reality requires a multipronged approach to treat and attempt to cure. This is when integrative medicine becomes key—and vital. In traditional medicine, it may seem like there are siloes across all the different areas—we divide medicine up into its various "departments" (e.g., heart disease vs. cancer vs. infectious disease vs. food allergy). But you might be surprised to learn that what we learn in one seemingly siloed area of medicine informs other areas. What we learn in researching Alzheimer's disease, for example, could have influential meaning on our understanding of immunology and related illnesses, food-related conditions among them. Even the development of novel therapies and vaccines for Covid-19 is currently revolutionizing medicine in ways we never thought possible.

This is why it's so important that we maintain an openness to new ideas and shifting paradigms in all of medicine and its disparate but related corners. Many other areas of medicine need to collaborate in solving the mystery of the modern allergy epidemic. This will take an interdisciplinary approach and includes insights from immunology, psychology/psychiatry, rheumatology, pulmonology, neurology, internal medicine, and microbiology (especially as it relates to the human micro-biome). At the end of the day, everything is a risk-benefit tradeoff. The more we can collect good data from all the relevant stakeholders, the better we can inform the best path forward.

The symptoms that we commonly associate with allergies—sneezing, eczema, runny nose, itchy eyes—are just the beginning. The prob-lem is that food allergies and their accomplices can impact any organ system and medicine is often segmented by system or organ. What's more, as you've learned by now, there are myriad overlapping symp-toms across the food allergy spectrum—from gastrointestinal issues to skin, oral, respiratory, cardiovascular, immunological, neurological, and psychological issues. It's a foregone conclusion: we need to look past the tried and tired clinical and research models. We cannot stay in our silos of specific disease conditions. The body is a complete, com-plex unit with everything having an impact on everything else, much like the world we live in. I do believe we will begin an era of collabo-ration and understanding, linked with new advancements in research and technology for a stronger and brighter future for all those living with a food condition.

Live Fearlessly

When I first began to even think about this book, my working title was *Food: Friend or Foe?* It seemed apt at the time. For people who live with conditions triggered by daily sustenance, the world—the palate of pos-sibilities—suddenly gets divided into two unequal halves: friends and foes. Good guys and bad guys. Sources of comfort and fear. As I began to collect my thoughts and ideas into a cohesive narrative while bringing in the science and all that I had learned as a researcher and doctor, the current title took shape. A life without fear of food is a life well-lived. We all deserve that. And it's possible when you shape food allergy and its relatives around the four-point directive: Identify and Empower; Treat; Manage and Prevent; and Thrive. This "prescription" is not always linear, for sometimes we manage and prevent at the same time, or we treat and then empower some more before re-identifying and treating again. As with so many things in life we experience, this prescriptive model is an endless continuum that we move through and around and within as needed. It's a framework for our choices, attitude, and illuminating the path forward. That path, by the way, is a bright one when we choose to walk it courageously.

Cody Skylar is a food allergy advocate and active member of FARE who is doing his part to change the world. As founder of Wander Meals, one of the world's first health-conscious, allergy-friendly meal delivery services, he hopes to create a world in which dietary restrictions and requirements do not define or control the life of anybody else. And he would know the importance of this mission: Cody suffers from severe anaphylactic food allergies to six of the top eight food allergens and was unable to speak until the age of four due to restrictions in his airways from allergic reactions. He summed up my broader view of things in a bold statement: "Life isn't about the birthday cake you may or may not be able to eat; it's about the breath you take to blow out your candles and make your wishes come true."

I couldn't have said it better myself. And finally, one of my favorite quotes by the great Maya Angelou: "Do the best you can until you know better. Then when you know better, do better." Through all the amazing work by clinicians, researchers, advocates, educators, and people like you, we know better every day.

Now go do your part. Find the area you can make a difference in and help us do better.

Breathe. Make your wishes come true. And thrive.

Fearless Facts

→ Although the entire spectrum of adverse food reactions will remain a major public health concern, the future for patients and their families is brighter than ever, with new technologies and therapies on the horizon.

→ Awareness is growing regarding the disparate burden that food-related conditions place on marginalized communities, and the tangible steps that can be taken to advance health equity for all.

→ Food allergy management is a job for every individual. Each one of us can fight for better food policy at local levels and organize in solidarity with regional and national patient advocacy organizations. With the power of a collective, societal force, we can usher in a reaction-free future and truly live fearlessly.

APPENDIX A

The Parent's Playbook

FEEDING A BABY FROM BREAST TO SOLIDS

There's a pervasive idea that a baby's digestive tract, or "gut," isn't mature enough to digest anything but breast milk until six months of age. A question I am often asked: Does this mean parents should wait to introduce solids until the six-month mark? My answer: Most babies will tell you when they are ready to start solids, somewhere between four and seven months. This is a very natural process. I recommend taking cues from the baby to assess whether they're ready for solid food. Are they sitting upright with good head control? Do they express interest in what you're eating? Can they take food from a spoon? If a child is at elevated risk for food allergy, though, the potential benefit of early introduction is also enhanced, and that potential benefit has to be weighed alongside the baby's feeding cues. Also, always work with your pediatrician and consider your family preferences. Breastfeeding exclusively until six months of age in low or moderate risk babies is absolutely fine. If the baby is at high risk, discuss with your pediatrician and allergist how to proceed but do begin the evaluation and introduction around four months. Studies find that early evaluation and possible early introduction may be most beneficial for high-risk infant.

Breast milk has long been known as the ideal nutrition for a baby; it's recommended by the American Academy of Pediatrics (AAP), which in 2012 reaffirmed its recommendation of *exclusive breastfeeding for about six months, followed by continued breastfeeding as complementary foods*

*are introduced, with continuation of breastfeeding for one year or longer
as mutually desired by mother and infant.* But breast milk's halo is not
only because of the nutrition it provides. Breast milk also plays a dynamic
role in the developing immune system, contributing to defense as well as
apparent hyperdefense in the form of allergy. The food allergen transfer
that naturally occurs during breastfeeding might confer a benefit of food
allergen, as this may be the first food exposure for the infant. Breast milk
is a complex immunologic liquid and is the most natural source of sustenance for babies.

The literature continues to grow regarding breast milk and food allergy; however, we have so much more to learn about how breast milk
impacts the development of food allergy. Breast milk is composed not only
of macro- and micronutrients but also of living cells, antibodies, and other
immunologically active agents, some of which fill immunological gaps in
the immature immune system. Breast milk composition is dynamic, changing as the baby develops and even altering with clinical changes, such as
in the face of infection. Bacteria are also present in human breast milk.
While the sources of some of these microorganisms are thought to include
a mother's skin and an infant's mouth and skin, plus the environment,
special immune cells in the mother can transport bacteria from her gut
through the lymphatic system and into her mammary glands, where the
bacteria are transferred into the breast milk. In addition, oligosaccharides
(also referred to as prebiotics)—a type of carbohydrate necessary for cellular functionality—are also present in breast milk and serve an important
role in the development of an infant's gut microbiota. This brings us to the
importance of supporting that microbiome I defined in Part 1.

I realize that exclusive breastfeeding in those first few months is not
realistic or even possible for some mothers for a variety of reasons, and
thankfully the infant formula market has improved immensely over the
years to try to mimic natural breast milk. A mother should never blame
herself for being unable to breastfeed exclusively or at all. Likewise, parents shouldn't blame themselves if their children develop food allergies
no matter how much they tried to avoid it.

This is a really important point, since no strategy for avoiding food allergy is perfect and recommendations continue to evolve as we learn more. There are some babies who will develop food allergies even if they are born vaginally, raised on a farm, are breastfed, require no antibiotics, and are given allergenic foods early. It's pointless for parents to speculate about the root cause of their child's allergies and cast blame.

Introducing Solid Foods: One at a Time

Food introduction is recommended by most pediatricians when the baby is developmentally ready, and this happens somewhere between four and six months for most babies. As mentioned, a baby should be able to sit up with little or no support, and show interest in food by opening his or her mouth when offered food. Babies ready for solid foods also try to grab food, toys, or other objects. Start with one food first. Examples include fortified baby cereal and pureed vegetable or fruit. Gradually offer new single-ingredient purees one at a time. Offer thin purees first and advance to mashed consistencies as a baby's palate adjusts to different textures. Then, you can progress by serving two-ingredient purees, such as meat mixed with a vegetable—mixing foods helps to increase diet diversity. Don't add any sugar or salt. Continue to provide breast milk or infant formula for the first year of life. Breast milk can be offered for as long as the mother and infant want.

Although most pediatricians recommend that families wait at least two days prior to the introduction of a new food to be able to monitor for an allergic reaction, this is not based on any solid scientific evidence and often makes it more difficult for parents to introduce a diverse assortment of foods in a timely fashion, while at the same time stressing them out with an overly medicalized approach. My advice, published by *JAMA* in August 2020, is to wait one to two days between each new food—one day for noncommon food allergens is probably just fine. Start by introducing a few fruit and vegetable purees, which can be mixed with fortified baby cereal. Once your baby has the hang of those, you can try some peanut products.

Remember, IgE-mediated food allergies typically occur within two hours of ingestion and over the majority are caused by the top nine allergens (peanut, tree nut, egg, milk, soy, wheat, finfish, shellfish, and sesame), whereas reactions to cereal, fruits, and vegetables are rare. Peanut products shouldn't be the first solid food a baby gets. To introduce other common allergens into your baby's diet, add such foods as yogurt (cow's milk), Cream of Wheat cereal (wheat), or a variety of nut butters (tree nuts). Eggs that are baked or hard-boiled (and thus extensively heated) are less likely to cause a reaction than eggs that are lightly cooked, such as when they're scrambled. So, try sneaking these foods into baked goods, such as homemade low-sugar muffins (using fruit puree instead of sugar) or hard-boiled egg pureed with a bit of water/breast milk/infant formula.

From what we know now, data suggest that the children who benefit the most from introduction of allergenic foods, such as peanut and egg, as early as four months are the children who are at highest risk of developing food allergy. For these children who are predisposed to allergic conditions, whose skin is likely to be damaged by eczema, it's best for their first exposure to allergenic foods to be through their mouth, as this promotes food tolerance. Remember the slogan: *Through the skin, allergies could begin. Through the diet, allergies can stay quiet.* It is also important to remember that many children with food allergies never had eczema and early introduction of food allergens is probably beneficial to all infants.

It is important to remember that the AAP recommendations to exclusively breastfeed for six months predates the LEAP study. Although this is still recommended, the AAP does recommend evaluation and earlier introduction of peanut products if the infant is at high risk. We also know from the EAT study, which was published in 2016, that introducing allergenic foods to babies at three months didn't disrupt breastfeeding between three and six months, so early introduction and breastfeeding can work together.

After the LEAP study was published, an expert panel was convened by the National Institute of Allergy and Infectious Diseases (NIAID) to develop guidelines for parents and physicians based on the new evidence that eating peanut foods early could protect against peanut allergy. AAP's 2019 guidance on early nutrition endorses the NIAID guidelines, which vary based on a baby's risk for peanut allergy. For babies at low risk, families can introduce age-appropriate peanut-containing foods when and how they like, so long as the peanut foods aren't choking hazards (see below). For babies who are at moderate risk for peanut allergy because they have mild or moderate eczema, NIAID recommends introduction of peanut foods around six months. For babies at highest risk, who have severe eczema, an egg allergy, or both, NIAID encourages parents to first have their baby tested to see whether the baby has already developed peanut allergy. If the baby isn't already allergic to peanut, they are better off eating age-appropriate peanut-containing foods as soon as they can, as the risk of developing a peanut allergy increases as the baby gets older.

2 Easy Ways to Introduce Peanut Foods to an Infant

1. Mix some smooth peanut butter with water, formula, breast milk, or pureed food, such as fruit and vegetables.
2. Use peanut-containing teething biscuits or peanut snacks.

For example, you can mix 2 teaspoons of smooth peanut butter into about 2 teaspoons of hot water, letting it cool down before feeding it. Alternatively mix the peanut butter into 3 tablespoons of fruit or vegetable puree. Start with a small amount of this mixture on the tip of a spoon, and then wait ten minutes for signs of a reaction. If that's tolerated, you can offer the rest of the serving. When we observed infants at our hospital who were brought in for allergic reactions, we found the majority had mild symptoms of hives or rash and vomiting, with trouble breathing and drop in blood pressure being less common. According to NIAID guidelines, feeding 2 grams of peanut protein (in the form of 2 teaspoons of peanut butter or peanut flour, or 21 pieces of Bamba peanut puffs, for instance) about three times per week is recommended, as was used in the LEAP study. As you increase intake of other nuts and nut butters, peanut intake may reduce a bit but try to give it to your infant as often as possible. The goal is to keep peanuts as a regular part of the diet.

To summarize the best recommendations to date, and based on the latest science, here's my advice, but please consult your child's pediatrician:

→ No dietary restrictions during pregnancy or breastfeeding (unless, of course, the mother has allergies or intolerances to certain foods)

→ If your baby has dry, red, inflamed skin, talk to your pediatrician right away. Use emollients and prescribed medications as needed to keep the skin intact and see a dermatologist if needed.

→ If your baby is diagnosed with severe eczema, make sure you talk to your baby's pediatrician early—around four months—to get your child tested for peanut allergy before introducing peanut into their diet. If necessary, your pediatrician may recommend you visit an allergist to conduct certain tests on your child. You should not delay in seeking out evaluation for peanut allergy. The absolute "window" to prevent food allergies is still not known, however delaying these could result in your child developing peanut allergy.

→ The recommendations for the introduction of egg or egg-containing products is similar: it should be around six months of age but not before four months of age. Recommendations include using the "cooked" forms of eggs and not raw or pasteurized-egg–containing products such as custards, homemade ice cream, mayonnaise, etc.

→ Do not delay the introduction of the other seven allergens such as cow's milk, tree nuts, soy, wheat, sesame, finfish, and shellfish. Once your baby is tolerating complementary foods you can try and introduce one new food at a time.

> Once your baby is tolerating these foods you should continue to introduce a diverse diet and continue to feed them these foods on a regular rotational basis.

I should add that genetics play a role in food allergy development but are not deterministic. A baby does not necessarily inherit peanut allergy from a parent with peanut allergy, or milk allergy when a sibling has milk allergy. Many children—the vast majority—with food allergy have no parental food allergy. Family history of food allergy, however, puts a baby at a slightly higher risk of developing a food allergy.

And I can't reiterate this enough: early food allergen introduction, specifically peanut introduction, has been repeatedly shown to decrease the risk of peanut allergy development especially in high-risk infants with severe eczema. Data for egg introduction and prevention of egg allergy and other foods are moving in the same direction and we will hopefully have additional data on this soon. And more broadly, studies on diet diversity indicate that eating a wider variety of healthy foods during infancy can lower the risk of developing food allergy.

A task force from the European Academy of Allergy and Clinical Immunology (EAACI) performed a systematic review of published studies and concluded that increased diet diversity may reduce the risk for food allergy. One study performed in multiple European countries and another one just in the UK reported that increased food diversity in the first year of life was associated with reduced food allergies in later childhood. Two important points can be taken from these studies: The UK study showed that for each additional food given by six months and for each additional food allergen given by twelve months, the chances of developing food allergy came down significantly.

The second important point we learned from diet diversity studies came from the European study, where a better infant diet characterized by intake of fish, yogurt, fruits, and vegetables was associated with more butyrate in the infant gut microbiome (a sign of a diverse and healthy gut microbiome) and less food allergies and other allergies in the child. The message is clear: We have to let the babies eat!

This does not mean that babies need to eat a lot of food by six months and eat every single possible food allergen by twelve months. What it does mean is that if you start weaning your baby before six months, don't just give baby rice and apple puree every day—give different fruits, vegetables, and grains. Enjoy this time with your infant, introducing them to some of your favorites. Just make sure not to give any food that could cause choking and do not give honey in the first year of life due to the potential for botulism. In terms of food allergens, it is important to introduce peanut-containing foods (smooth peanut butter diluted with water, breast milk, or formula) early on to mitigate the risk of developing peanut allergy and continue to introduce other foods as part of the family diet. The golden rule is: Once you have introduced a food allergen, do keep it in the diet regularly.

My colleague Dr. Carina Venter is an allergy specialist dietitian at the University of Colorado/Children's Hospital Colorado. She works diligently to understand how nutrition, microbiome, immunology, and genetics relate to food allergy prevention and treatment. As one of the founding members and past chair of the International Network for Diet and Nutrition in Allergy, she has helped to create a home for dietitians interested in researching food allergy, and stresses the importance of understanding maternal and infant nutrition in the treatment and prevention of food allergy.

In June 2020, Dr. Venter published a study showing that increased diet diversity in a cohort of almost one thousand infants decreased their likelihood of developing food allergy. She also helped conduct a systematic review that explored the association between diet diversity and allergy outcomes in infancy and childhood. Based on their findings, she and her colleagues also suggest that diet diversity in infancy may be associated with reduced allergy outcomes, and are working to determine clear guidelines for appropriate diet diversity in infants.

Dr. Venter is pleased that nutrition is finally getting its rightful place in the world of food allergy, and the role of nutrition in allergic disorders is finally being extensively studied. She notes, "Nutrition does not only support the immune system; it also offers a modifiable factor for prevention and treatment benefits. I truly believe that immonutrition may provide many of the answers we need."

I am grateful for the opportunity to work alongside Dr. Venter to address some of these issues. I particularly look forward to translating our research endeavors into educational activities worldwide in the future. This will provide us the opportunity to define the best way to introduce foods to infants and prevent allergic disease through research, while decreasing the medicalization and promoting this natural life experience for babies to learn to eat and explore their world.

THE EDUCATION OF FOOD ALLERGY IN PUBLIC SETTINGS: SCHOOL PREPAREDNESS

Food allergy preparedness is especially important in schools, where children spend so much of their young lives under the care and supervision of their teachers and school staff. About 18 percent of children with food allergy have experienced an allergic reaction at school, and as many as a quarter (25 percent) of first-time allergic reactions occur in school due to young children trying foods for the first time or accidental ingestion. With this in mind, it's important to ensure students with food allergy, their teachers, and their peers are well informed about how to maintain a safe environment as they navigate through early childhood, elementary school, middle school, high school, and beyond.

First and foremost, it's important to understand the different inclusive and protective food allergy policies in effect at each school. About ten years ago, I worked to help improve the guidelines for managing life-threatening food allergies in Illinois schools. At the time, schools were unauthorized to keep an emergency supply of epinephrine for children who did not have a diagnosed food allergy or autoinjector, and further, school health personnel were not permitted to administer any lifesaving medication to these children due to fear of liability. But after a young Chicago eighth grader died of anaphylaxis at a school celebration, the Chicago Public Schools (CPS) district committed to never have this happen again, and in 2012, the Illinois attorney general officially passed the School Access to Emergency Epinephrine Act. CPS became the first large urban school district in the country with this lifesaving medication widely and readily available for all students and staff. It was incredible to be part of this experience and today, forty-nine US states either have laws/guidelines allowing or requiring schools to stock epinephrine or actually require schools to stock epinephrine to keep their children safe—and the fiftieth is on its way.

In addition to school epinephrine policies, many schools adopt varying policies to address food allergies, such as providing nut-free foods, encouraging families not to bring products with allergens, designating allergen-free lunch tables, and banning outside food from coming into the school. I'm so thankful for the strides made in school systems to make the environment as safe as possible for students with food allergy. It's immensely important to educate faculty, staff, and students, regardless of the allergen-free policies in place. Now, I'll walk you through each stage of the school spectrum with tips and tools to keep in mind for food allergy safety and preparedness.

Early Childhood

Sending a child with food allergy to preschool or daycare may be the first time that they are placed in the care of someone else. As young children may not yet be able to articulate how they are feeling or may not be aware of their symptoms, it's important to educate their teachers on how to recognize the signs and symptoms of reactions and how to intervene appropriately. Ways to facilitate this process are to notify the schools of the child's allergies as early as possible, including their diagnosis, type of allergies, and reaction history, and to provide teachers with the child's food allergy emergency action plan (explained more on page 274). In addition, bringing all of their necessary medications to school and keeping an open dialogue with the teachers to share information and resources are incredibly beneficial—for example, letting the teacher know how and when to use epinephrine in case of an emergency, and discussing the typical language or signs used when your child experiences a reaction, so they can feel prepared.

Our team recently created helpful educational videos for early childhood professionals, parents, and students to facilitate these conversations and educate this population so everyone feels empowered to care for children with food allergy. The videos can be found on our website: https://www.feinberg.northwestern.edu/sites/cfaar/resources/video-library.html.

Elementary School/Middle School

As children reach elementary school age, it's important to discuss sharing foods and smart, safe ways to eat during lunchtime or in the cafeteria. Students at this age are beginning to become more independent and social, so equipping them with the confidence and knowledge of what they can and cannot share is critical during this stage. Encouraging teachers to provide non-food-related items for celebrations throughout the school year to avoid any accidental ingestions will also be helpful to make for a fun, safe, and stress-free environment. As students start to move into middle school, they are also more likely to take more of an independent role with their food allergy. More students are allowed to self-carry their epinephrine autoinjectors, so ensure students have their epinephrine in an accessible place and know how and when to use it.

Moreover, make sure they have a physician-signed permission form to self-carry/self-inject if necessary. Students with food allergy are their own most powerful advocates; practice epinephrine use with them and educate their friends and teachers so they can provide support as well!

Again, always make sure the school nurse or teacher has an action plan on file, and can care for students appropriately and effectively.

High School

As students reach high school age, they have often taken a more independent role in management and sometimes engage in more risk-taking behaviors around their food allergy. In a study my team conducted in 2016, we aimed to understand the behaviors and factors that influence teens to take risks with their food allergy. We found that 13 percent of students do not always carry an epinephrine autoinjector, and many reported eating packaged foods with precautionary allergen labeling (PAL) that contained their most severe allergens as potential ingredients. In addition, when they were asked whether their classmates would know what to do in case of a food allergy emergency, only about 11 percent indicated their peers would know how to intervene. However, those who had school support (teacher, friend, school nurse awareness of their food allergy) were less likely to partake in risky behaviors. Overall, students indicated that more public awareness of food allergy and better support from their schools are needed to help them feel more comfortable in the school setting. However, these adolescents also indicated that living with food allergy has benefited them in many ways. For instance, it has helped them feel more responsible, become a better advocate for themselves and others, appreciate and offer help to others with special needs, and make healthier food selections for themselves.

During this school stage, it's important to encourage these behaviors and ensure there are support systems in place at their schools to make them feel safe and empowered to care for their food allergy appropriately. To aid conversation across all of these age groups, my team has created three peer-to-peer food allergy educational videos aimed to increase awareness of food allergy and early identification of anaphylaxis symptoms. The goal of these videos is to empower students to be advocates for themselves in and out of the classroom, and help teachers by providing them with useful FAQs and resources to get the discussion started. To access these videos, go to: https://www.feinberg.northwestern .edu/sites/cfaar/resources/video-library.html.

College/University

As students transition into college life, they will be leaving their established support systems at home and will have to start independently managing their food allergy on campus. Although many new systems are in place to accommodate college students with food allergy and other food-related conditions, there are a few key tips to keep in mind to prepare for this stage. When students are applying for colleges and going on college visits, it is an ideal time to start asking questions about accommodations on campus. Although food allergy accommodations won't be the sole factor for selecting a college, understanding who the stakeholders on campus are and any systems in place are helpful for determining safety when students are in the dining halls, in the dorms, at group events, and beyond. Contacting the campus disability services (if applicable), the dining staff, and housing contacts can help to answer questions about safety protocols and important considerations before getting started on their college journeys.

Colleges are still in the early stages of distinguishing standardized safety measures for students with food-related conditions, and we've done work to understand what supports are still needed on college campuses to make students feel safe and accommodated. In a 2018 study, we interviewed students with food allergy and key stakeholders on a college campus to figure out the key areas for improvement. The stakeholders indicated that the transition to college for students with food allergy would be improved by providing support for (1) notification of others in the student's campus network about food allergy; (2) establishing clearly defined roles/responsibilities; and (3) increasing campus awareness of food allergy signs, symptoms, and lethality. Through this feedback, we created a prototype for a food allergy toolkit called "Spotlight on

Campus Food Allergies" with different interventions to improve the college experience with food allergy. The interventions included tools for before orientation, ideas for improvement in the dining halls, support when joining a club or sports team, and proper food-labeling protocols for student outings. We're hoping to bring these ideas to life on college campuses across the nation.

To this end, we've also been surveying students about any reactions—and causes—they've experienced in the dining halls, as well as what they believe can be done better on campus to improve awareness and accommodations. Through this survey, we will create an educational video to be shown at college orientations to start the conversation as early as possible, and equip students and their peers with the tools they need to have a successful and safe college experience.

Emergency Action Plans and Medical Alert Jewelry

As mentioned earlier, an asset that all patients with IgE-mediated food allergy should have is a written emergency action plan and clear communication with others who may have to help intervene during a reaction at school or work. These written plans should be easy to read and follow, aimed at treating symptoms of a reaction without needing an advanced degree. Doses of medications should also be listed on the emergency action plan. Sample emergency action plans are available in both English and Spanish. The ones I like best have been created by the American Academy of Pediatrics (AAP), as well as by FARE. These are easily downloadable online; see Resources.

Some schools, local school boards, and states may have their own emergency action plans. When it comes to school-aged children, it's important that families collaborate with the school nurses, school nutrition services (to requests dietary substitutions), and their allergists. School nurses are key partners as they have the necessary skills and leadership to create and implement food allergy policies, train and educate school staff, bring awareness to the school community, and respond to allergic emergencies. Also, they are aware of the resources and culture of their schools, in addition to the school staff that they work with. They are instrumental in the management of anaphylaxis for both those with known allergies and those whose allergies are unknown to the school. Unfortunately, full-time school nurses are not available in all schools.

Regardless of the presence of a full-time school nurse, the faculty and staff need to be trained, and where there's no school nurse, staff training becomes even more critical. In cases when a school nurse is unavailable, staff will need to be trained to implement student-specific and schoolwide food allergy management strategies. All school staff should be trained to recognize allergic reactions and anaphylaxis and know their role in their school's food allergy emergency protocol. In most states, select staff with appropriate training may be trained to administer epinephrine to those without a known history of allergic reactions when the school nurse is not immediately available. It is also important to educate a child's friends. Again, we found that one of the biggest factors in decreased risk taking for teens with food allergy was peer support. If friends know and support their friends, they always do better.

It goes without saying that it's critical to establish open communication and seek support when there are unreasonable expectations on the part of the family or school, or when school allergy management strategies are either not effectively keeping the student safe or are overly restrictive and impacting quality of life, the ability to learn, or the other students. To that end, I encourage anyone who is at risk for a serious reaction to consider medical alert jewelry, including bracelets or necklace tags, as these can be extremely helpful for first responders if someone is found unconscious. They can also be helpful for individuals who may not be able to articulate that they are having a reaction. Imagine dining alone in a restaurant when a bad reaction strikes from accidental ingestion of an ingredient to which you're highly allergic. Within minutes, you can barely talk, let alone breathe. If someone nearby can know immediately what's going on, it just might save your life. Now, that's an extreme example but it makes a good point.

APPENDIX B

Resources

Medical Organizations: National

American Academy of Allergy, Asthma, and Immunology (AAAAI)	https://www.aaaai.org/
American Academy of Pediatrics (AAP)	https://www.aap.org/
American College of Allergy, Asthma, & Immunology (ACAAI)	https://acaai.org/

Medical Organizations: International

Allergy & Anaphylaxis Australia	www.allergyfacts.org.au
Allergy Care India	www.allergycareindia.org
Allergy New Zealand	www.allergy.org.nz
Allergy UK	www.allergyuk.org
Anaphylaxis Campaign	www.anaphylaxis.org.uk
Canadian Society of Allergy and Clinical Immunology (CSACI)	https://csaci.ca/
European Academy of Allergy and Clinical Immunology	https://www.eaaci.org/
Food Allergy Canada	https://foodallergycanada.ca/
Fundacion S.O.S. Alergia	www.sosalergia.org
Swiss Institute of Allergy and Asthma Research (SIAF)	www.siaf.uzh.ch
World Allergy Organization	www.worldallergy.org

Key Government Agencies

Centers for Disease Control and Prevention (CDC)	cdc.gov
ClinicalTrials.gov	www.clinicaltrials.gov
Immune Tolerance Network (ITN)	www.immunetolerance.org
National Institutes of Health: National Institute of Allergy and Infectious Diseases	https://www.niaid.nih.gov/
US Department of Agriculture	https://www.usda.gov/
US Food and Drug Administration	www.fda.gov

Hospitals/Centers

Asthma, Allergy & Food Allergy Centers, St. Louis, Missouri	https://aafacenters.com/about-us/dr-warrier/
Center for Food Allergy & Asthma Research (CFAAR)	https://www.feinberg.northwestern.edu/sites/cfaar/
Children's Hospital Colorado	https://www.childrenscolorado.org
FARE (Food Allergy Research & Education)	https://www.foodallergy.org/resources/fare-clinical-network-centers-distinction
Gores Family Allergy Center at Children's Hospital Los Angeles	https://www.chla.org/gores-family-allergy-center
Jaffe Food Allergy Institute, Icahn School of Medicine at Mount Sinai	https://icahn.mssm.edu/research/jaffe
King's College Hospital, UK	https://www.kch.nhs.uk/
Mary H. Weiser Food Allergy Center	https://medicine.umich.edu/dept/food-allergy-center
Murdoch Children's Research Institute Centre for Food and Allergy Research, Australia	https://www.mcri.edu.au/research/centres/centre-food-and-allergy-research
Northwest Asthma & Allergy Center	https://www.nwasthma.com/
Northwestern Medicine Allergy and Immunology Division	https://www.nm.org/conditions-and-care-areas/allergy-and-immunology

Texas Children's Hospital Food Allergy Program, Baylor College of Medicine	https://www.texaschildrens.org/departments/food-allergy-program
University of Colorado Division of Allergy, Asthma, and Clinical Immunology	https://medschool.cuanschutz.edu/clinical-immunology
University of Nebraska–Lincoln, Food Allergy Research and Resource Program	https://farrp.unl.edu/

National Advocacy Organizations

Allergy Advocacy Association	https://allergyadvocacyassociation.org/
Allergy & Asthma Network (AAN)	https://www.allergyasthmanetwork.org/
Allergy Home	www.allergyhome.org
Allergy Strong	https://allergystrong.com/
American Partnership for Eosinophilic Disorders	https://apfed.org
Asthma and Allergy Foundation of America (AAFA)	https://www.aafa.org/
British Society for Allergy & Clinical Immunology	https://bsaci.org
Campaign Urging Research for Eosinophilic Diseases (CURED)	https://curedfoundation.org
Celiac Disease Foundation	https://celiac.org/
Eat Right: Academy of Nutrition and Dietetics	https://www.eatright.org/
Food Allergy & Anaphylaxis Connection Team (FAACT)	https://www.foodallergyawareness.org/
Food Allergy Fund	https://foodallergyfund.org/
FARE (Food Allergy Research & Education)	https://www.foodallergy.org/
Food Equality Initiative	https://foodequalityinitiative.org/
FPIES Foundation	https://fpiesfoundation.org/
International Food Protein–Induced Enterocolitis Syndrome Association	https://fpies.org/

| Kids with Food Allergies—A Division of the Asthma and Allergy Foundation of America | https://www.kidswithfoodallergies.org/ |

Family Foundations/Influencers

Allergic Traveler	https://www.allergictraveler.net/
Allergy Travels	https://www.facebook.com/groups/allergytravels/
Allison Rose Foundation	https://www.allisonrosefoundation.org/
Elijah-Alavi Foundation	https://www.elijahalavifoundation.org/
Enchanting Family Vacations	https://www.enchantingfamilyvacations.net/
Equal Eats	https://www.equaleats.com/
Food Allergy Pros	https://foodallergypros.com/
Food Allergy Treatment Talk Facebook Group	https://www.facebook.com/chewtheFATT/
Light It Teal	https://www.lightitteal.org/
Love for Giovanni Foundation	https://www.loveforgiovanni.org/
Natalie Giorgi Sunshine Foundation	https://nateam.org/
No Nut Traveler	http://nonuttraveler.com/
Red Sneakers for Oakley	https://www.redsneakers.org/

Support Groups

Celiac Disease Support Groups	https://nationalceliac.org/celiac-disease-support-groups/
FARE (Food Allergy Research & Education)	https://www.foodallergyawareness.org/education/support-groups/food-allergy-support-groups/
Food Allergy Research & Education	https://www.foodallergy.org/living-food-allergies/join-community/find-support-group

Food Allergy Support and Education Program (FASE)	https://www.luriechildrens.org/en/specialties-conditions/food-allergy-support-education-program/
FPIES Support Forum	https://thefpiesfoundation.hoop.la/
Friends Helping Friends Food Allergy Support Group	https://www.facebook.com/groups/1448583488780077
Gluten-Free Living	https://www.glutenfreeliving.com/
Kids with Food Allergies Forum (main)	https://community.kidswithfoodallergies.org/forum/main_forum
Mothers of Children Having Allergies (MOCHA)	https://mochallergies.org/
No Nuts Moms Group (NNMG), Facebook	https://www.facebook.com/groups/nnmgforum/
No Nuts Moms Group (support group website)	https://nonutsmomsgroup.weebly.com/
Parents of Children with Allergies (POCA) of DuPage	http://pocaofdupage.org/index.html
SupportGroups.com: Food Allergy	http://food-allergy.supportgroups.com

Apps/Tools

Alerje	http://alerje.com/
Allergy Amulet	http://www.allergyamulet.com/
Allergy Assist	https://allergyassistprogram.com/
Allergy Eats	https://www.allergyeats.com/
Allergy Force	https://www.allergyforce.com/
Belay	https://www.webelay.com/
Gluten Free Passport	https://glutenfreepassport.com
Nima	https://nimasensor.com/
Picknic	https://picknic.app/
Smart Label	http://www.smartlabel.org/
Snack Safely	https://snacksafely.com/at-home/
Spokin	https://www.spokin.com/

APPENDIX C
Sample Food Log

U SE THE FOLLOWING AS A TEMPLATE FOR YOUR FOOD DIARY ENTRIES. YOU can keep a journal or notebook of your meals and snacks on paper or simply make your entries on a computer in a file you create. The goal is to record the contents of your meals and snacks, any reactions you experience, and the timing—when the reactions occur, how soon after you eat do symptoms develop, and how those symptoms progress and change over time. The goal is to find patterns. Sharing the diary with your doctor and/or dietitian will help you figure out the cause of your problems.

Do not hesitate to document symptoms that may not seem related to food, such as a headache, joint pain, dizziness, skin problems, or mood changes. And don't forget to include beverages, cooking oils, and additions to meals, such as condiments, garnishes, or other toppings. List brands where appropriate. Describe type of food (e.g., processed, restaurant, home cooked, etc.). Be as comprehensive as possible, including any medications taken, plus vitamins and supplements. Although you're not counting calories, you may want to include serving sizes. Also note any lifestyle or other factors that may be related, such as having a reaction to a meal after vigorous exercise or managing/treating another condition simultaneously (e.g., infection, injury, menstrual cycle, acute stress). Contact with animals, latex, pollen, perfumes, mold, fresh paint, and so on, should also be noted. You can even go so far as to write down the weather and season. The more detailed you can be, the better.

DATE	FOOD OR LIQUID	AMOUNT	TIME CONSUMED	TIME OF REACTION

SYMPTOMS	OTHER REMARKS

ACKNOWLEDGMENTS

THE LIST OF THOSE TO WHOM I FEEL GRATEFUL COULD FILL A BOOK TWICE this size. This book belongs to so many experts and families whose knowledge and experiences made this all possible.

First, to Bonnie Solow for making that initial call to me years ago when we commenced this important journey and for supporting me every step of the way with unending resolve when we had to reposition the goalposts. And for introducing me to my co-author Kristin: you are so talented and an incredible partner, and I am beyond proud of what we've accomplished.

To our patient and insightful editor, Renée Sedliar, whose guidance and feedback kept me on task and open to new ideas about content and organizational flow, as well as the rest of the Hachette Go team: Mary Ann Naples, Michelle Aielli, Michael Barrs, Alison Dalafave, Lauren Rosenthal, and Zachary Polendo. And to the production team: Amber Morris, Linda Mark, Iris Bass, and Zan Ceeley.

To my "work family," this book is our success. It feels like a dream to think about how far we've come. To create our Center for Food Allergy and Asthma Research (CFAAR) has been one of my proudest accomplishments, and this book underlines the magnitude of our work to improve the lives of adults, children, and their families with food conditions. To those on the team who helped bring this book to life: Madeleine Kanaley, Dr. Christopher Warren, and Justin Zaslavsky, thank you for your dedication to our mission.

I must also thank the experts in the field who read, researched, and helped polish the manuscript, working tirelessly to make sure we presented the information accurately: Drs. Allan Bock, Aaron Donnell, Sai Nimmagadda, Carina Venter, and Manoj Warrier. Your passion for this work is palpable and knowledge unmatched.

In addition, I want to thank the experts in allergy, GI, dermatology, nutrition, pediatrics, research, advocacy, policy, and the families living with food conditions every day who read and edited sections specific to their expertise. Dr. Katrina Allen, Dr. Sakina Bajowala, Dr. Helen Brough, Emily Brown, Dave and Denise Bunning, Dr. Christina Ciaccio, Dr. George du Toit, Lisa Gable, Dr. Gideon Lack, Dr. Peter Lio, Dr. Lisa Lombard, Dr. Kari Nadeau, Dr. Cathryn Nagler, Dr. Anna Nowak-Wegrzyn, Dr. Amy Paller, Dr. Hugh Sampson, Dan and Fritzie Shinohara, Dr. Scott Sicherer, Cody Skylar, Dr. Pooja Tandon, Caryn and Susan Tatelli, Dr. Stephen Taylor, Jamison ("JJ") Vulopas, Tonya Winders, and Dr. Josh Wechsler: Thank you all for sharing your incredible stories and for your expert feedback. I feel so fortunate for our collaborations throughout the years and am honored to work alongside each and every one of you.

To those partners that allow our team to achieve our goals: from public sponsors like the National Institute of Allergy and Infectious Diseases to foundations to the NGOs and advocacy organizations who share our vision of a world in which everyone can experience "Food Without Fear."

To my husband Tarun—thanks for your constant support, honesty, and encouragement; my kids, Rohan and Riya, thank you for always cheerleading my work and for making it so personal; my parents and sister Raina for building the foundation on which I stand; and to all my additional family and friends for always listening and being there.

I am hopeful for the future as there is so much research happening in this field. The more we learn and discover, the more we realize we need to learn and discover. Finally, I am eternally grateful for all who read this book and develop a better understanding of their food condition. In the words of one of my favorite poets, Maya Angelou: "Do the best you can until you know better. Then when you know better, do better."

NOTES

THE FOLLOWING IS A PARTIAL LIST OF SCIENTIFIC PAPERS AND OTHER REFER-
ences that you might find helpful in learning more about some of the
ideas and concepts expressed in this book. To have included every possible citation would have taken up hundreds of pages, but I have cited the
particular studies mentioned in the book. For more, I invite you to explore
the National Library of Medicine online (at https://pubmed.ncbi.nlm.nih
.gov/) and visit my faculty page at https://www.feinberg.northwestern
.edu to access a full list of my publications. FoodAllergy.org also main-
tains a large database of resources you might find helpful and that can
open the door for further inquiry.

INTRODUCTION: Welcome to Food Freedom

R. S. Gupta, Elizabeth E. Springston, Manoj R. Warrier, et al., "The Prevalence, Severity, and Distribution of Childhood Food Allergy in the United
States," *Pediatrics* 128, no. 1 (July 2011): e9–e17, https://doi.org/10.1542/peds
.2011-0204.

R. S. Gupta, C. M. Warren, B. M. Smith, et al., "Prevalence and Severity
of Food Allergies Among US Adults," *JAMA Network Open* 2, no. 1 (2019):
e185630, https://doi.org/10.1001/jamanetworkopen.2018.5630.

CHAPTER 1: Body Backlash: The Surprising Rise of Reactions
to Food in the 21st Century and the Search for Answers

American Academy of Allergy, Asthma & Immunology (AAAAI), "Allergy
Statistics," https://www.aaaai.org/about-aaaai/newsroom/allergy-statistics.

The Centers for Disease Control and Prevention, www.cdc.gov.

Kathleen C. Chambers, "Conditioned Taste Aversions," *World Journal of Otorhinolaryngology—Head & Neck Surgery* 4, no. 1 (March 2018): 92–100.

Food Allergy Research and Education (FARE), "Facts and Statistics," https://www.foodallergy.org/resources/facts-and-statistics.

R. S. Gupta, D. Holdford, L. Bilaver, et al., "The Economic Impact of Childhood Food Allergy in the United States," *JAMA Pediatrics* 167, no. 11 (2013): 1026–1031, https://doi.org/10.1001/jamapediatrics.2013.2376.

R. S. Gupta, Elizabeth E. Springston, Manoj R. Warrier, et al., "The Prevalence, Severity, and Distribution of Childhood Food Allergy in the United States," *Pediatrics* 128, no. 1 (July 2011): e9–e17, https://doi.org/10.1542/peds.2011-0204.

R. S. Gupta, C. M. Warren, B. M. Smith, et al., "Prevalence and Severity of Food Allergies Among US Adults," *JAMA Network Open* 2, no. 1 (2019): e185630, https://doi.org/10.1001/jamanetworkopen.2018.5630.

R. S. Gupta, C. M. Warren, B. M. Smith, et al., "The Public Health Impact of Parent-Reported Childhood Food Allergies in the United States," *Pediatrics* 142, no. 6 (December 2018): e20181235, Epub November 19, 2018, https://doi.org/10.1542/peds.2018–1235, erratum in *Pediatrics* 143, no. 3 (March 2019): PMID: 30455345; PMCID: PMC6317772.

National Institute of Allergy and Infectious Diseases (NIAID), https://www.niaid.nih.gov/.

JJ Vulopas, Riya Jain, Suzy Brauer, et al., *The Class That Can: Food Allergies* (Chicago: Citizens That Can, LLC, 2019).

Kathleen Y. Wang, Juhee Lee, Antonella Cianferoni, et al., "Food Protein-Induced Enterocolitis Syndrome Food Challenges: Experience from a Large Referral Center," *Journal of Allergy and Clinical Immunology Practice* 7, no. 2 (February 2018): 444–450, Epub September 20, 2018, https://doi.org/10.1016/j.jaip.2018.09.009.

CHAPTER 2: "Allergies" Are Not All Created Equal:
Anatomy of Immune-Based Reactions vs. Masqueraders on the Spectrum

Shaffiq Idris Alkhatib, "Woman with Allergy Dies After Eating Prawns," *Straits Times* (August 22, 2017), https://www.straitstimes.com/singapore/courts-crime/woman-with-allergy-dies-after-eating-prawns.

American Academy of Allergy, Asthma & Immunology (AAAAI), www.aaaai.org.

David Bloom, "What We Learned from the George Hodgkiss Tragedy," SackSafely.com (February 27, 2018), https://snacksafely.com/2018/02/what-we-learned-from-the-george-hodgkiss-tragedy/.

Geoffrey Carlson and Christopher Coop, "Pollen Food Allergy Syndrome (PFAS): A Review of Current Available Literature," *Annals of Allery, Asthma, and Immunology* 123, no. 4 (July 2019): 359–365, https://doi.org/10.1016/j .anai.2019.07.022.

Wyatt W. Decker, Ronna L. Campbell, Veena Manivannan, et al., "The Etiology and Incidence of Anaphylaxis in Rochester, Minnesota: A Report from the Rochester Epidemiology Project," *Journal of Allergy and Clinical Immunology* 122, no. 6 (December 2008): 1161–1165, Epub November 6, 2008, https://doi.org/10.1016/j.jaci.2008.09.043.

R. S. Gupta, ed., *Pediatric Food Allergy: A Clinical Guide* (New York: Springer International Publishing, 2020).

J. Molina-Infante, A. M. Schoepfer, A. J. Lucendo, and E. S. Dellon, "Eosinophilic Esophagitis: What Can We Learn from Crohn's Disease?" *United European Gastroenterology Journal* 5, no. 6 (2017): 762–772, https://doi.org /10.1177/2050640616672953.

I. Reche, G. D'Orta, N. Mladenov, et al., "Deposition Rates of Viruses and Bacteria Above the Atmospheric Boundary Layer," *ISME Journal* 12, no.1154–1162 (2018), https://doi.org/10.1038/s41396-017-0042-4.

Nicole Smith, "Florida Teen Dies Following Severe Allergic Reaction to Peanut," *Allergic Living*, June 29, 2018, https://www.allergicliving.com/2018 /06/29/florida-teen-dies-following-severe-allergic-reaction-to-peanut/.

CHAPTER 3: The Genome, Epigenome, Microbiome, and Risk for Allergies: Why Our Body Can Become Confused, Bewildered, and Inflamed

Katrina J. Allen, Jennifer J. Koplin, Anne-Louise Ponsonby, et al., "Vitamin D Insufficiency Is Associated with Challenge-Proven Food Allergy in Infants," *Journal of Allergy and Clinical Immunology* 131, no., 4 (April 2013): 1109–1116, Epub February 27, 2013, https://doi.org/10.1016/j.jaci.2013.01 .017.

American Academy of Pediatrics, Committee on Nutrition, "Hypoallergenic Infant Formulas," *Pediatrics* 106, 2, pt. 1 (August 2000): 346–349.

Karin Amrein, Mario Scherkl, Magdalena Hoffmann, et al., "Vitamin D Deficiency 2.0: An Update on the Current Status Worldwide," *European Journal of Clinical Nutrition* 74, no. 11 (November 2020): 1498–1513, Epub January 20, 2020, https://doi.org/10.1038/s41430-020-0558-y.

"Anaphylaxis Hypothesis," *Annals of Allergy, Asthma & Immunology* 103, no. 6 (December 2009): 488–495, https://doi.org/10.1016/S1081-1206 (10)60265-7.

Yuka Asai, Aida Eslami, C. Dorien van Ginkel, et al., "Genome-Wide Association Study and Meta-analysis in Multiple Populations Identifies New Loci for Peanut Allergy and Establishes C11orf30/EMSY as a Genetic Risk Factor for Food Allergy," *Journal of Allergy and Clinical Immunology* 141, no. 3 (March 2018): 991–1001, Epub October 10, 2017, https://doi.org/10 .1016/j.jaci.2017.09.015.

Sara Benedé, Ana Belen Blázquez, David Chiang, et al., "The Rise of Food Allergy: Environmental Factors and Emerging Treatments," *EBioMedicine* 7 (May 2016): 27–34, Epub April 16, 2016, https://doi.org/10.1016/j.ebiom.2016 .04.012.

Helen A. Brough, Kari C. Nadeau, Sayantani B. Sindher, et al., "Epicutaneous Sensitization in the Development of Food Allergy: What Is the Evidence and How Can This Be Prevented?" *Allergy* 75, no. 9 (September 2020): 2185– 2205, Epub May 18, 2020, https://doi.org/10.1111/all.14304.

Ewen Callaway, "C-section Babies Are Missing Key Microbes," *Nature*, September 2019, https://doi.org/10.1038/d41586-019-02807-x.

Carlos A. Camargo Jr., Sunday Clark, Michael S. Kaplan, et al., "Regional Differences in EpiPen Prescriptions in the United States: The Potential Role of Vitamin D," *Journal of Allergy and Clinical Immunology* 120, no. 1 (July 2007): 131–136, Epub June 7, 2007, https://doi.org/10.1016/j.jaci.2007.03.049.

C. E. Ciaccio, "Modulating the Microbiome: The Future of Allergy Therapeutics?" *Annals of Allergy, Asthma & Immunology* 122, no. 3 (2019): 233– 235, Epub December 12, 2018, https://doi.org/10.1016/j.anai.2018.12.006.

Debra De Silva, Susanne Halken, Chris Singh, et al., "Preventing Food Allergy in Infancy and Childhood: Systematic Review of Randomized Controlled Trials," *Pediatric Allergy and Immunology* 31, no. 7 (October 2020): 813–826, Epub June 18, 2020, https://doi.org/10.1111/pai.13273.

George du Toit, Graham Roberts, Peter H. Sayre, et al., "Identifying Infants at High Risk of Peanut Allergy: The Learning Early About Peanut Allergy (LEAP) Screening Study," *Journal of Allergy and Clinical Immunology* 131, no. 1 (January 2013): 135–143, Epub November 19, 2012, https://doi.org/10 .1016/j.jaci.2012.09.015.

George du Toit, Graham Roberts, Peter H. Sayre, et al., "Randomized Trial of Peanut Consumption in Infants at Risk for Peanut Allergy," *New England Journal of Medicine* 372, no. 9 (February 2015): 803–813, Epub February 23, 2015, https://doi.org/10.1056/NEJMoa1414850.

George du Toit, Ru-Xin Foong, and Gideon Lack, "Prevention of Food Allergy—Early Dietary Interventions," *Allergology International* 65, no. 4 (October 2016): 370–377, https://doi.org/10.1016/j.alit.2016.08.001, Epub September 9, 2016.

Tove Fall, Cecilia Lundholm, Anne K. Örtqvist, et al., "Early Exposure to Dogs and Farm Animals and the Risk of Childhood Asthma," *JAMA Pediatrics* 169, no. 11 (November 2015): e153219, Epub November 2, 2015, https://doi .org/10.1001/jamapediatrics.2015.3219.

David M. Fleischer, Jonathan M. Spergel, Amal H. Assa'ad, and Jacque line A. Pongracic, "Primary Prevention of Allergic Disease Through Nutritional Interventions," *Journal of Allergy and Clinical Immunology in Practice* 1, no. 1 (January 2013): 29–36, Epub November 22, 2012, https://doi.org /10.1016/j.jaip.2012.09.003.

Jelle Folkerts, Ralph Stadhouders, Frank A. Redegeld, et al., "Effect of Dietary Fiber and Metabolites on Mast Cell Activation and Mast Cell-Associated Diseases," *Frontiers in Immunology* 9 (May 2018): 1067, eCollection 2018, https://doi.org/10.3389/fimmu.2018.01067.

P. D. Gluckman and M. A. Hanson, "The Developmental Origins of Health and Disease." In *Early Life Origins of Health and Disease. Advances in Experimental Medicine and Biology*, eds. E. M. Wintour and J. A. Owens, vol. 573 (Boston: Springer, 2006), https://doi.org/10.1007/0-387-32632 -4_1.

Frank R. Greer, Scott H. Sicherer, A. Wesley Burks, Committee on Nutrition; Section on Allergy and Immunology, "The Effects of Early Nutritional Interventions on the Development of Atopic Disease in Infants and Children: The Role of Maternal Dietary Restriction, Breastfeeding, Hydrolyzed Formulas, and Timing of Introduction of Allergenic Complementary Foods," *Pediatrics* 143, no. 4 (April 2019): e20190281, Epub March 18, 2019, https://doi .org/10.1542/peds.2019-0281.

R. S. Gupta, Anne Marie Singh, Madeline Walkner, et al., "Hygiene Factors Associated with Childhood Food Allergy and Asthma," *Allergy and Asthma Proceedings* 37, no. 6 (November 2016): e140–e146, https://doi.org/10.2500 /aap.2016.37.3988.

R. S. Gupta, C. M. Warren, B. M. Smith, et al., "Prevalence and Severity of Food Allergies Among US Adults," *JAMA Network Open* 2, no. 1 (2019): e185630, https://doi.org/10.1001/jamanetworkopen.2018.5630.

R. S. Gupta, Xingyou Zhang, Elizabeth E. Springston, et al., "The Association Between Community Crime and Childhood Asthma Prevalence in Chicago," *Annals of Allergy, Asthma & Immunology* 104, no. 4 (April 2010): 299–306, https://doi.org/10.1016/j.anai.2009.11.047.

Lauren A. Hesser, Jeffrey Hubbell, and Cathryn Nagler, "Optimizing Bacteriotherapy to Prevent or Treat Food Allergy," *Journal of Immunology* 204, suppl. 1 (May 2020): 158.20.

Michael F. Holick, "Vitamin D Deficiency," *New England Journal of Medicine* 357, no. 3 (July 2007): 266–281, https://doi.org/10.1056/NEJMra070553.

Onyinye I. Iweala and Cathryn R. Nagler, "The Microbiome and Food Allergy," *Annual Review of Immunology* 37 (April 2019): 377–403, https://doi .org/10.1146/annurev-immunol-042718-041621.

W. Karmaus and C. Botezan, "Does a Higher Number of Siblings Protect Against the Development of Allergy and Asthma? A Review," *Journal of Epidemiology and Community Health* 56, no. 3 (March 2002): 209–217, https://doi.org/10.1136/jech.56.3.209.

G. Lack, "Epidemiologic Risks for Food Allergy," *Journal of Allergy and Clinical Immunology* 121, no. 6 (June 2008): 1331–1336, https://doi.org/10.1016/j.jaci.2008.04.032.

Gideon Lack and Deborah E. Fox, "Peanut Allergy," *Lancet* 352, no. 9129 (August 29, 1998): 741, https://doi.org/10.1016/S0140-6736(05)60863-X.

LEAP Study, http://www.leapstudy.com/.

London Allergy Care and Knowledge, "Research," http://www.london allergy.com/research-and-development/.

Mirembe Mandy and Moffat Nyirenda, "Developmental Origins of Health and Disease: The Relevance to Developing Nations," *International Health* 10, no. 2 (March 2018): 66–70, https://doi.org/10.1093/inthealth/ihy006.

David Martino, Thanh Dang, Alexandra Sexton-Oates, et al., "Blood DNA Methylation Biomarkers Predict Clinical Reactivity in Food-sensitized Infants," *Journal of Allergy and Clinical Immunology* 143, no. 5 (May 2015): 1319–1328.e1–12, Epub February 10, 2015, https://doi.org/10.1016/j.jaci.2014.12.1933.

Emily C. McGowan, Roger Peng, Päivi M Salo, et al., "Cockroach, Dust Mite, and Shrimp Sensitization Correlations in the National Health and Nutrition Examination Survey," *Annals of Allergy, Asthma & Immunology* 122, no. 5 (May 2019): 536–538.e1, Epub February 23, 2019, https://doi.org/10.1016/j.anai.2019.02.015.

Niki Mitselou, Jenny Hallberg, Olof Stephansson, et al., "Cesarean Delivery, Preterm Birth, and Risk of Food Allergy: Nationwide Swedish Cohort Study of More than 1 Million Children," *Journal of Allergy and Clinical Immunology* 142, no. 5 (November 2018): 1510–1514.e2, Epub September 10, 2018, https://doi.org/10.1016/j.jaci.2018.06.044.

Raymond James Mullins and Carlos A. Camargo, "Latitude, Sunlight, Vitamin D, and Childhood Food Allergy/Anaphylaxis," *Current Allergy and Asthma Reports* 12, no. 1 (February 2012): 64–71, https://doi.org/10.1007/s11882-011-0230-7.

Raymond James Mullins, Sunday Clark, and Carlos A. Camargo Jr., "Regional Variation in Epinephrine Autoinjector Prescriptions in Australia: More Evidence for the Vitamin D-anaphylaxis hypothesis," *Ann Allergy Asthma Immunol* 103, no. 6 (December 2009): 488–495, https://doi:10.1016/S1081-1206(10)60265-7.

Rathish Nair and Arun Maseeh, "Vitamin D. The 'Sunshine' Vitamin," *Journal of Pharmacology and Pharmacotherapeutics* 3, no. 2 (April 2012): 118–126, https://doi.org/10.4103/0976-500X.95506.

National Academies of Sciences, Engineering, and Medicine; Health and Medicine Division; Food and Nutrition Board; Committee on Food Allergies: Global Burden, Causes, Treatment, Prevention, and Public Policy, "Finding a Path to Safety in Food Allergy: Assessment of the Global Burden, Causes, Prevention, Management, and Public Policy," eds. M. P. Oria and V. A. Stallings (Washington, DC: National Academies Press, November 30, 2016), PMID: 28609025.

National Institute of Allergy and Infectious Diseases (NIAID), "Food Allergy," https://www.niaid.nih.gov/diseases-conditions/food-allergy.

Kathrin Negele, Joachim Heinrich, Michael Borte, et al., "Mode of Delivery and Development of Atopic Disease During the First 2 Years of Life," *Pediatric Allergy and Immunology* 15, no. 1 (February 2004): 48–54, https://doi.org/10.1046/j.0905-6157.2003.00101.x.

Nicholas J. Osborne, Obioha C. Ukoumunne, Melissa Wake, and Katrina J. Allen, "Prevalence of Eczema and Food Allergy Is Associated with Latitude in Australia," *Journal of Allergy and Clinical Immunology* 129, no. 3 (March 2012): 865–867, Epub February 2, 2012, https://doi.org/10.1016/j.jaci.2012.01.037.

Evangelia Papathoma, Maria Triga, Sotirios Fouzas, and Gabriel Dimitriou, "Cesarean Section Delivery and Development of Food Allergy and Atopic Dermatitis in Early Childhood," *Pediatric Allergy and Immunology* 27, no. 4 (June 2016): 419–424, https://doi.org/10.1111/pai.12552.

K. Robbins, M. Jacobs, A. Ramos, et al., "Prenatal Food Allergen Avoidance Practices for Food Allergy Prevention," *Annals of Allergy, Asthma, and Immunology* 121, no. 5 (November 2018): S55–S56, https://doi.org/10.1016/j.anai.2018.09.180.

Daniel E. Roth, Steven A. Abrams, John Aloia, et al., "Global Prevalence and Disease Burden of Vitamin D Deficiency: A Roadmap for Action in Low- and Middle-Income Countries," *Annals of the New York Academy of Sciences* 1430, no. 1 (October 2018): 44–79, Epub September 18, 2018, https://doi.org/10.1111/nyas.13968.

Scott H. Sicherer, Katrina Allen, Gideon Lack, et al., "Critical Issues in Food Allergy: A National Academies Consensus Report," *Pediatrics* 140, no. 2 (August 2017): e20170194, https://doi.org/10.1542/peds.2017-0194.

Scott H. Sicherer and Hugh A. Sampson, "Food Allergy: A Review and Update on Epidemiology, Pathogenesis, Diagnosis, Prevention, and Management," *Journal of Allergy and Clinical Immunology* 141, no. 1 (January 2018): 41–58, Epub November 21, 2017, https://doi.org/10.1016/j.jaci.2017.11.003.

J. I. Silverberg, E. L. Simpson, H. G. Durkin, and R. Joks, "Prevalence of Allergic Disease in Foreign-Born American Children," *JAMA Pediatrics* 167, no. 6 (2013): 554–560, https://doi.org/10.1001/jamapediatrics.2013.1319.

Anne Marie Singh, "Barriers in Food Allergy Prevention," *Science Translational Medicine* 16 (March 2016): 330EC45.

Joy L. Snyder and Guha Krishnaswamy, "Autoimmune Progesterone Dermatitis and Its Manifestation as Anaphylaxis: A Case Report and Literature Review," *Annals of Allergy, Asthma & Immunology* 90, no. 5 (May 2003): 469–477; quiz 477, 571, https://doi.org/10.1016/S1081-1206(10)61838-8.

Andrew T. Stefka, Taylor Feehley, Prabhanshu Tripathi, et al., "Commensal Bacteria Protect Against Food Allergen Sensitization," *Proceedings of the National Academy of Sciences* (USA) 111, no. 36 (September 2014): 13145–13150, https://doi.org/10.1073/pnas.1412008111.

D. P. Strachan, "Hay Fever, Hygiene, and Household Size," *BMJ* 299, no. 6710 (November 1989): 1259–1260, https://doi.org/10.1136/bmj.299.6710.1259.

Aleena Syed, Marco A. Garcia, Shu-Chen Lyu, et al., "Peanut Oral Immunotherapy Results in Increased Antigen-Induced Treg Function and Hypomethylation of FOXP3," *Journal of Allergy and Clinical Immunology* 133, no. 2 (February 2014): 500–510, https://doi.org/10.1016/j.jaci.2013.12.1037.

United European Gastroenterology, "Half of All Commonly Used Drugs Profoundly Affecting the Gut Microbiome, Warn Experts," MedicalXPress .com, October 23, 2019, https://medicalxpress.com/news/2019-10-commonly -drugs-profoundly-affecting-gut.html.

Arnau Vich Vila, Valerie Collij, Serena Sanna, et al., "Impact of Commonly Used Drugs on the Composition and Metabolic Function of the Gut Microbiota," *Nature Communications* 11, no. 1 (January 2020): 362, https://doi.org /10.1038/s41467-019-14177-z.

John Wei-Liang Tan, Carolina Valerio, Elizabeth H. Barnes, et al., "A Randomized Trial of Egg Introduction from 4 Months of Age in Infants at Risk for Egg Allergy," *Journal of Allergy and Clinical Immunology* 139, no. 5 (May 2017): 1621–1628.e8, Epub October 11, 2016, https://doi.org/10.1016/j.jaci .2016.08.035.

Tamar Weinberger and Scott Sicherer, "Current Perspectives on Tree Nut Allergy: A Review," *Journal of Asthma and Allergy* 11 (2018): 41–51, Epub March 26, 2019, https://doi.org/10.2147/JAA.S141636.

E. Kenneth Weir, Thenappan Thenappan, Maneesh Bhargava, and Yingjie Chen, "Does Vitamin D Deficiency Increase the Severity of COVID-19?" *Clinical Medicine* (London) 20, no. 4 (July 2020): e107–e108, Epub June 5, 2020, https://doi.org/10.7861/clinmed.2020-0301.

Yuxia Zhang, Fiona Collier, Gaetano Naselli, et al., "Cord Blood Monocyte-Derived Inflammatory Cytokines Suppress IL-2 and Induce Nonclassic

'T(II)2-Type' Immunity Associated with Development of Food Allergy," *Science Translational Medicine* 8, no. 321 (January 2016): 321ra8, https://doi.org /10.1126/scitranslmed.aad4322.

CHAPTER 4: Inflammation, Allergies, Autoimmune Diseases, and Other Ailments: The Hidden Connections of Immune Dysfunction

Azza Abdel-Gadir, Emmanuel Stephen-Victor, Georg K. Gerber, et al., "Microbiota Therapy Acts via a Regulatory T Cell MyD88/RORγt Pathway to Suppress Food Allergy," *Nature Medicine* 25, no. 7 (July 2019): 1164–1174, Epub June 24, 2019, https://doi.org/10.1038/s41591-019-0461-z.

Rok Son Choung and Nicholas J. Talley, "Food Allergy and Intolerance in IBS," *Gastroenterology and Hepatology* (NY) 2, no. 10 (October 2006): 756–760.

A. Fritscher-Ravens, Detlef Schuppan, Mark Ellrichmann, et al., "Confocal Endomicroscopy Shows Food-Associated Changes in the Intestinal Mucosa of Patients with Irritable Bowel Syndrome," *Gastroenterology* 147, no. 5 (2014): 1012, Epub July 30, 2014, https://doi.org/10.1053/j.gastro.2014.07.046.

Pradipta Ghosh, Lee Swanson, Ibrahim M. Sayed, et al., "The Stress Polarity Signaling (SPS) Pathway Serves as a Marker and a Target in the Leaky Gut Barrier: Implications in Aging and Cancer," *Life Science Alliance* 3, no. 3 (February 2020): e201900481, https://doi.org/10.26508/lsa.201900481.

Uday C. Ghoshal, Ratnakar Shukla, and Ujjala Ghoshal, "Small Intestinal Bacterial Overgrowth and Irritable Bowel Syndrome: A Bridge between Functional Organic Dichotomy," *Gut and Liver* 11, no. 2 (March 2017): 196–208, https://doi.org/10.5009/gnl16126.

R. S. Gupta, C. M. Warren, B. M. Smith, et al., "The Public Health Impact of Parent-Reported Childhood Food Allergies in the United States," *Pediatrics* 142, no. 6 (December 2018): e20181235, https://doi.org/10.1542/peds .2018-1235, Epub November 19, 2018; erratum in: *Pediatrics* 2143, no. 3 (March 2019): PMID: 30455345; PMCID: PMC6317772.

R. S. Gupta, C. M. Warren, B. M. Smith, et al., "Prevalence and Severity of Food Allergies Among US Adults," *JAMA Network Open* 2, no. 1 (2019): e185630, https://doi.org/10.1001/jamanetworkopen.2018.5630.

Mamidipudi Thirumala Krishna, Anuradhaa Subramanian, Nicola J. Adderley, et al., "Allergic Diseases and Long Term Risk of Autoimmune Disorders: Longitudinal Cohort Study and Cluster Analysis," *European Respiratory Journal* 54, no. 5 (January 2019): 1900476, https://doi.org/10.1183/13993003 .00476-2019.

Lan Lin, Timothy P. Moran, Bin Peng, et al., "Walnut Antigens Can Trigger Autoantibody Development in Patients with Pemphigus Vulgaris Through a

'Hit-and-Run' Mechanism," *Journal of Allergy and Clinical Immunology* 144, no. 3 (September 2019): 720–728.e4, Epub May 6, 2019, https://doi.org /10.1016/j.jaci.2019.04.020.

Mayo Clinic, "Food Sensitivities May Affect Gut Barrier Function," November 12, 2016, https://www.mayoclinic.org/medical-professionals/digestive -diseases/news/food-sensitivities-may-affect-gut-barrier-function/mac -20429973.

Qinghui Mu, Jay Kirby, Christopher M. Reilly, and Xin M. Luo, "Leaky Gut as a Danger Signal for Autoimmune Diseases," *Frontiers in Immunology* 8 (May 2017): 598, eCollection 2017, https://doi.org/10.3389/fimmu.2017.00598.

Matthew A. Odenwald and Jerrold R. Turner, "The Intestinal Epithelial Barrier: A Therapeutic Target?" *Nat Rev Gastroenterol Hepatol* 14, no. 1 (January 2017): 9–21, Epub November 16, 2016, https://doi.org/10.1038/nrgastro .2016.169.

Ayesha Shah, Nicholas J. Talley, Mike Jones, et al., "Small Intestinal Bacterial Overgrowth in Irritable Bowel Syndrome: A Systematic Review and Meta-Analysis of Case-Control Studies," *American Journal of Gastroenterology* 115, no. 2 (February 2020): 190–201, https://doi.org/10.14309/ajg.0000000000000 504.

Caroline J. Tuck, Jessica R. Biesiekierski, Peter Schmid-Grendelmeier, and Daniel Pohl, "Food Intolerances," *Nutrients* 11, no. 7 (July 2019): 1684, https://doi.org/10.3390/nu11071684.

M. I. Vazquez Roque, Michael Camilleri, Thomas Smyrk, et al., "A Controlled Trial of Gluten-Free Diet in Patients with Irritable Bowel Syndrome-Diarrhea: Effects on Bowel Frequency and Intestinal Function," *Gastroenterology* 144, no. 5 (2013): 903, Epub January 25, 2013, https://doi.org/10.1053/j .gastro.2013.01.049.

CHAPTER 5: Caution: May Contain . . . : A Cornucopia of Confusion

Donald R. Davis, Melvin D. Epp, and Hugh D. Riordan, "Changes in USDA Food Composition Data for 43 Garden Crops, 1950 to 1999," *Journal of the American College of Nutrition* 23, no. 6 (December 2004): 669–682, https:// doi.org/10.1080/07315724.2004.10719409.

Mária Ercsey-Ravasz, Zoltán Toroczkai, Zoltán Lakner, and József Baranyi, "Complexity of the International Agro-food Trade Network and Its Impact on Food Safety," *PLoS One* 7, no. 5 (2012): e37810, Epub May 31, 2012, https:// doi.org/ 10.1371/journal.pone.0037810.

Food and Drug Administration, "Agricultural Biotechnology," https:// www.fda.gov/food/consumers/agricultural-biotechnology?utm_source=google &utm_medium=search&utm_campaign=feedyourmind2020.

Food and Drug Administration, "Food Allergen Labeling and Consumer Protection Act of 2004 (FALCPA)," https://www.fda.gov/food/food-allergensgluten-free-guidance-documents-regulatory-information/food-allergen-labeling-and-consumer-protection-act-2004-falcpa.

Food and Drug Administration, "Food Safety Modernization Act (FSMA)," https://www.fda.gov/food/guidance-regulation-food-and-dietary-supplements/food-safety-modernization-act-fsma.

Food and Drug Administration, "Full Text of the Food Safety Modernization Act (FSMA)," https://www.fda.gov/food/food-safety-modernization-act-fsma/full-text-food-safety-modernization-act-fsma.

Food and Drug Administration, "How GMOs Are Regulated for Food and Plant Safety in the United States," https://www.fda.gov/food/agricultural-biotechnology/how-gmos-are-regulated-food-and-plant-safety-united-states.

Kate E. C. Grimshaw, Graham Roberts, Anna Selby, et al., "Risk Factors for Hen's Egg Allergy in Europe: EuroPrevall Birth Cohort," *Journal of Allergy and Clinical Immunology: In Practice* 8 no. 4 (April 2020): 1341-1348.e5, Epub December 14, 2019, https://doi.org/10.1016/j.jaip.2019.11.040.

R. Gupta, Madeleine Kanaley, Olivia Negris, et al., "Understanding Precautionary Allergen Labeling (PAL) Preferences Among Food Allergy Stakeholders," *Journal of Allergy and Clinical Immunology in Practice* (September 2020): S2213–2198(20)31000-X, https://doi.org/10.1016/j.jaip.2020.09.022.

R. S. Gupta, S. L. Taylor, J. L. Baumert, et al., "Economic Factors Impacting Food Allergen Management: Perspectives from the Food Industry," *Journal of Food Protection* 80, no. 10 (October 2017): 1719–1725, https://doi.org/10.4315/0362-028X.JFP-17-060.

Alison Hewitt, "Bait and Switch: UCLA Study Finds Fish Fraud Runs Rampant," January 11, 2017, UCLA Newsroom, https://newsroom.ucla.edu/releases/bait-and-switch-ucla-study-finds-fish-fraud-runs-rampant.

Elham Hossny, Motohiro Ebisawa, Yehia El-Gamal, et al., "Challenges of Managing Food Allergy in the Developing World," *World Allergy Organization Journal* 12, no. 11 (December 2019): 100089, eCollection November 2019, https://doi.org/10.1016/j.waojou.2019.100089.

Institute of Medicine (US), "Improving Food Safety Through a One Health Approach: Workshop Summary" (Washington, DC: National Academies Press, 2012), PMID: 23230579; see A5: "Overview of the Global Food System: Changes Over Time/Space and Lessons for Future Food Safety" by Will Hueston and Anni McLeod.

Kyunguk Jeong, Jihyun Kim, Kangmo Ahn, et al., "Age-Based Causes and Clinical Characteristics of Immediate-Type Food Allergy in Korean Children," *Allergy, Asthma & Immunology Research* 9, no. 5 (September 2017): 423–430, https://doi.org/10.4168/aair.2017.9.5.423.

Jialing Jiang, Chitra Dinakar, Jamie L. Fierstein, et al., "Food Allergy Among Asian Indian Immigrants in the United States," *Journal of Allergy and Clinical Immunology in Practice* 8, no. 5 (May 2020): 1740–1742, Epub January 7, 2020, https://doi.org/10.1016/j.jaip.2019.12.026.

Shaun Kennedy, "University Research in Food Safety and Food Defense," Presentation for the National Center for Food Protection and Defense, National Academy of Sciences, September 29, 2009, https://sites.nationalacademies.org /cs/groups/pgasite/documents/webpage/pga_053570.pdf.

Robert E. Levin, Flora-Glad C. Ekezie, and Da-Wen Sun, "DNA-Based Technique: Polymerase Chain Reaction (PCR)," in *Modern Techniques for Food Authentication* 2nd. ed., ed. Da-Wen Sun (San Diego, CA: Academic Press, 2018): 527–616, https://doi.org/10.1016/B978-0-12-814264-6.00014-1.

Mahboobeh Mahdavinia, Susan R. Fox, Bridget M. Smith, et al., "Racial Differences in Food Allergy Phenotype and Health Care Utilization Among US Children," *Journal of Allergy and Clinical Immunology in Practice* 5, no. 2 (March–Apr 2017): 352–357.e1, https://doi.org/10.1016/j.jaip.2016.10.006, Epub November 23, 2016.

Mary Jane Marchisotto, Laurie Harada, Opal Kamdar, et al., "Food Allergen Labeling and Purchasing Habits in the United States and Canada," *Journal of Allergy and Clinical Immunology in Practice* 5, no. 2 (March–April 2017): 345–351.e2, Epub November 3, 2016, https://doi.org/10.1016/j.jaip.2016.09.020.

Robin J. Marles, "Mineral Nutrient Composition of Vegetables, Fruits and Grains: The Context of Reports of Apparent Historical Declines," *Journal of Food Composition and Analysis* 56 (March 2017): 93–103, https://doi.org/10 .1016/j.jfca.2016.11.012.

M. Panjari, J. J. Koplin, S. C. Dharmage, et al., "Nut Allergy Prevalence and Differences Between Asian-Born Children and Australian-Born Children of Asian Descent: A State-Wide Survey of Children at Primary School Entry in Victoria, Australia," *Clinical and Experimental Allergy* 46, no. 4 (April 2016): 602–609, https://doi.org/10.1111/cea.12699.

Michael T. Roberts and Whitney Turk, White Paper: *The Pursuit of Food Authenticity: Recommended Legal & Policy Strategies to Eradicate Economically Motivated Adulteration (Food Fraud)*, UCLA School of Law, March 28, 2017, https://law.ucla.edu/sites/default/files/PDFs/Publications/_RES_PUB %20fraud%20report.pdf.

A. A. Schoemaker, A. B. Sprikkelman, K. E. Grimshaw, et al., "Incidence and Natural History of Challenge-proven Cow's Milk Allergy in European Children—EuroPrevall Birth Cohort," *Allergy* 70, no. 8 (August 2015): 963–972, Epub May 18, 2015, https://doi.org/10.1111/all.12630.

Jonathan I. Silverberg, Eric L. Simpson, Helen G. Durkin, and Rauno Joks, "Prevalence of Allergic Disease in Foreign-born American Children,"

JAMA Pediatrics 167, no. 6 (June 2013): 554–560, https://doi.org/10.1001/jamapediatrics.2013.1319.

Elizabeth Huiwen Tham and Donald Y. M. Leung, "How Different Parts of the World Provide New Insights into Food Allergy," *Allergy, Asthma & Immunology Research* 10, no. 4 (July 2018): 290–299, https://doi.org/10.4168/aair.2018.10.4.290.

Ondulla T. Toomer, Elliot Sanders, Thien C. Vu, et al., "Potential Transfer of Peanut and/or Soy Proteins from Poultry Feed to the Meat and/or Eggs Produced," *ACS Omega* 5, no. 2 (January 2020): 1080–1085, eCollection January 21, 2020, https://doi.org/10.1021/acsomega.9b03218.

US Department of Agriculture, "Organic 101: What the USDA Organic Label Means," https://www.usda.gov/media/blog/2012/03/22/organic-101-what-usda-organic-label-means#:~:text=Produce%20can%20be%20called%20organic,most%20synthetic%20fertilizers%20and%20pesticides.

Helen T. Wang, Christopher M. Warren, Ruchi S. Gupta, and Carla M. Davis, "Prevalence and Characteristics of Shellfish Allergy in the Pediatric Population of the United States," *Journal of Allergy and Clinical Immunology in Practice* 8, no. 4 (April 2020): 1359–1370.e2, Epub January 7, 2020, https://doi.org/10.1016/j.jaip.2019.12.027.

Christopher M. Warren, Avneet S. Chadha, Scott H. Sicherer, et al., "Prevalence and Severity of Sesame Allergy in the United States," *JAMA Network Open* 2, no. 8 (August 2019): e199144, https://doi.org/10.1001/jamanetworkopen.2019.9144.

Christopher M. Warren, Paul J. Turner, R. Sharon Chinthrajah, and Ruchi S. Gupta, "Advancing Food Allergy Through Epidemiology: Understanding and Addressing Disparities in Food Allergy Management and Outcomes," *Journal of Allergy and Clinical Immunology in Practice* S2213-2198(20)31114-4 (October 2020), https://doi.org/10.1016/j.jaip.2020.09.064, published online ahead of print.

C. M. Warren, J. Jiang, and Ruchi Gupta, "Epidemiology and Burden of Food Allergy," *Current Allergy and Asthma Reports* 20, no. 2 (February 2020): 6, https://doi.org/10.1007/s11882-020-0898-7.

P. Xepapadaki, A. Fiocchi, L. Grabenhenrich, et al., "Incidence and Natural History of Hen's Egg Allergy in the First 2 Years of Life—The EuroPrevall Birth Cohort Study," *Allergy* 71, no. 3 (March 2016): 350–357, Epub December 22, 2015, https://doi.org/10.1111/all.12801.

CHAPTER 6: Identify and Empower:
How to Make Sense of Imperfect Testing Methods

American Academy of Allergy, Asthma & Immunology (AAAAI), "Food Allergy Testing," https://acaai.org/allergies/types/food-allergies/testing.

Lucy A. Bilaver, Avneet S. Chadha, Priyam Doshi, et al., "Economic Burden of Food Allergy: A Systematic Review," *Annals of Allergy, Asthma & Immunology* 122, no. 4 (April 2019): 373–380.e1, Epub January 28, 2019, https://doi.org /10.1016/j.anai.2019.01.014.

Lucy A. Bilaver, Kristen M. Kester, Bridget M. Smith, and Ruchi S. Gupta, "Socioeconomic Disparities in the Economic Impact of Childhood Food Allergy," *Pediatrics* 137, no. 5 (May 2016): e20153678, https://doi.org/10.1542 /peds.2015-3678.

John H. Dunlop and Corinne A. Keet, "Epidemiology of Food Allergy," *Immunology and Allergy Clinics of North America* 38, no. 1 (February 2018): 13–25, Epub October 26, 2017, https://doi.org/10.1016/j.iac.2017.09.002.

Food Allergy Research and Education (FARE), "Blood Tests," https://www .foodallergy.org/resources/blood-tests#:~:text=Your%20allergist%20may %20order%20additional,to%20the%20food%20being%20tested.

R. Gupta, D. Holdford, L. Bilaver, et al., "The Economic Impact of Childhood Food Allergy in the United States," *JAMA Pediatrics* 167, no. 11 (2013): 1026–1031, https://doi.org/10.1001/jamapediatrics.2013.2376.

Johns Hopkins Medicine, "Warning: Food Allergy Blood Tests Sometimes Unreliable," July 17, 2007, https://www.hopkinsmedicine.org/news/media /releases/warning_food_allergy_blood_tests_sometimes_unreliable.

C. D. May, "Objective Clinical and Laboratory Studies of Immediate Hypersensitivity Reactions to Foods in Asthmatic Children," *Journal of Clinical Immunology* 58, no. 4 (October 1976): 500–515.

Javier Molina-Infante, Ángel Arias, Javier Alcedo, et al., "Step-up Empiric Elimination Diet for Pediatric and Adult Eosinophilic Esophagitis: The 2-4-6 Study," *Journal of Allergy and Clinical Immunology* 141, no. 4 (April 2018): 1365–1372, Epub October 23, 2017, https://doi.org/10.1016/j.jaci .2017.08.038.

Nicolaos Nicolaou, Maryam Poorafshar, Clare Murray, et al., "Allergy or Tolerance in Children Sensitized to Peanut: Prevalence and Differentiation Using Component-Resolved Diagnostics," *Journal of Allergy and Clinical Immunology* 125, no. 1 (January 2010): 191–197.e1–13, https://doi.org/10 .1016/j.jaci.2009.10.008.

Richard C. Nolan, Peter Richmond, Susan L. Prescott, et al., "Skin Prick Testing Predicts Peanut Challenge Outcome in Previously Allergic or Sensitized Children with Low Serum Peanut-Specific IgE Antibody Concentration," *Pediatric Allergy and Immunology* 18, no. 3 (May 2007): 224–230, https:// doi.org/10.1111/j.1399-3038.2007.00519.x.

Scott H. Sicherer, Katrina Allen, Gideon Lack, et al., "Critical Issues in Food Allergy: A National Academies Consensus Report," *Pediatrics* 140, no. 2 (August 2017): e20170194, https://doi.org/10.1542/peds.2017-0194.

David R. Stukus, Erin Kempe, Amy Leber, et al., "Use of Food Allergy Panels by Pediatric Care Providers Compared with Allergists," *Pediatrics* 138, no. 6 (December 2016): e20161602, https://doi.org/10.1542/peds.2016-1602.

Robert A. Wood, Nathan Segall, Staffan Ahlstedt, and P. Brock Williams, "Accuracy of IgE Antibody Laboratory Results," *Annals of Allergy, Asthma & Immunology* 99, no. 1 (July 2007): 34–41, https://doi.org/10.1016/S1081-1206(10)60618-7.

CHAPTER 7: Treatment: Current and Cutting-Edge Therapies

Philippe Begin, R. Sharon Chinthrajah, and Kari C. Nadeau, "Oral Immunotherapy for the Treatment of Food Allergy," *Human Vaccines & Immunotherapeutics* 10, no. 8 (August 2014): 2295–2302, https://doi.org/10.4161/hv.29233.

A. Wesley Burks, Stacie M. Jones, Robert A. Wood, et al., "Oral Immunotherapy for Treatment of Egg Allergy in Children," *New England Journal of Medicine* 367, no. 3 (July 2012): 233–243, https://doi.org/10.1056/NEJMoa1200435.

Food and Drug Administration, "Palforzia," https://www.fda.gov/vaccines-blood-biologics/allergenics/palforzia.

R. Gupta, D. Holdford, L. Bilaver, et al., "The Economic Impact of Childhood Food Allergy in the United States," *JAMA Pediatrics* 167, no. 11 (2013): 1026–1031, https://doi.org/10.1001/jamapediatrics.2013.2376.

Hannah M. Kansen, Thuy-My Le, Yolanda Meijer, et al., "The Impact of Oral Food Challenges for Food Allergy on Quality of Life: A Systematic Review," *Pediatric Allergy and Immunology* 29, no. 5 (August 2018): 527–537, Epub May 16, 2018, https://doi.org/10.1111/pai.12905.

Xiu-Min Li, "Treatment of Asthma and Food Allergy with Herbal Interventions from Traditional Chinese Medicine," *Mount Sinai Journal of Medicine* 78, no. 5 (September–October 2011): 697–716, https://doi.org/10.1002/msj.20294.

Chunrong Lin, Ivan T. Lee, Vanitha Sampath, et al., "Combining Anti-IgE with Oral Immunotherapy," *Pediatric Allergy and Immunology* 28, no. 7 (November 2017): 619–627, Epub September 7, 2017, https://doi.org/10.1111/pai.12767.

A. Martorell, E. Alonso, L. Echeverría, et al., "Oral Immunotherapy for Food Allergy: A Spanish Guideline. Immunotherapy Egg and Milk Spanish Guide" (ITEMS Guide). Part I: "Cow Milk and Egg Oral Immunotherapy: Introduction, Methodology, Rationale, Current State, Indications, Contraindications, and Oral Immunotherapy Build-Up Phase," *Journal of Investigational Allergology and Clinical Immunology* 27, no. 4 (2017): 225–237, https://doi.org/10.18176/jiaci.0177.

Zoë Slote Morris, Steven Wooding, and Jonathan Grant, "The Answer Is 17 Years, What Is the Question: Understanding Time Lags in Translational Research," *Journal of the Royal Society of Medicine* 104, no. 12 (December 2011): 510–520, https://doi.org/10.1258/jrsm.2011.110180.

G. Patriarca, E. Nucera, C. Roncallo, et al., "Oral Desensitizing Treatment in Food Allergy: Clinical and Immunological Results," *Alimentary Pharmacology & Therapeutics* 17, no. 3 (2003): 459–465.

C. Patriarca, A. Romano, A. Venuti, et al., "Oral Specific Hyposensitization in the Management of Patients Allergic to Food," *Allergologia et Immunopathologia* (Madrid) 12, no. 4 (1984): 275–281.

G. Patriarca, D. Schiavino, E. Nucera, et al., "Food Allergy in Children: Results of a Standardized Protocol for Oral Desensitization," *Hepatogastroenterology* 45, no. 19 (January–February 1998): 52–58.

Alfred T. Schofield, "A Case of Egg Poisoning," *Lancet* 171, no. 4410 (March 1908): 716, https://doi.org/10.1016/S0140-6736(00)67313-0.

Stanford T. Shulman, "Clemens von Pirquet: A Remarkable Life and Career," *Journal of the Pediatric Infectious Diseases Society* 6, no. 4 (November 2017): 376–379, https://doi.org/10.1093/jpids/piw063.

Scott H. Sicherer and Hugh A. Sampson, "Food Allergy," *Journal of Allergy and Clinical Immunology* 125, 2 suppl. 2 (February 2010): S116–S125, https://doi.org/10.1016/j.jaci.2009.08.028, Epub December 29, 2009.

Matthew Smith, "The Art of Medicine: Another Person's Poison," *Lancet* 384 (December 2014): 2019–2020.

Yamini V. Virkud and Brian P. Vickery, "Advances in Immunotherapy for Food Allergy," *Discovery Medicine* 14, no. 76 (September 2012): 159–165.

Julie Wang and Xiu-Min Li, "Chinese Herbal Therapy for the Treatment of Food Allergy," *Current Allergy and Asthma Reports* 12, no. 4 (August 2012): 332–338, https://doi.org/10.1007/s11882-012-0265-4.

CHAPTER 8: Manage and Prevent: Setting the Stage for a Reaction-Free Life

Katrina J. Allen, Jennifer J. Koplin, Anne-Louise Ponsonby, et al., "Vitamin D Insufficiency Is Associated with Challenge-Proven Food Allergy in Infants," *Journal of Allergy and Clinical Immunology* 131, no., 4 (April 2013): 1109–1116, 1116.e1-6, Epub February 27, 2013, https://doi.org/10.1016/j.jaci.2013.01.017.

Syed Hasan Arshad, Belinda Bateman, Alireza Sadeghnejad, et al., "Prevention of Allergic Disease During Childhood by Allergen Avoidance: The Isle of Wight Prevention Study," *Journal of Allergy and Clinical Immunology* 119, no. 2 (February 2007): 307–313, https://doi.org/10.1016/j.jaci.2006.12.621.

Meghan B. Azad, Theodore Konya, Heather Maughan, et al., "Gut Microbiota of Healthy Canadian Infants: Profiles by Mode of Delivery and Infant Diet at 4 Months," *Canadian Medical Association Journal* 185, no. 5 (March 2013): 385–394, Epub February 11, 2013, https://doi.org/10.1503/cmaj.121189.

Luciana Besedovsky, Tanja Lange, Monika Haack, et al., "The Sleep-Immune Crosstalk in Health and Disease," *Physiological Reviews* 99, no. 3 (July 2019): 1325–1380, https://doi.org/10.1152/physrev.00010.2018.

Ewen Callaway, "Scientists Swab C-Section Babies with Mothers' Microbes," *Nature News*, Springer Nature (February 1, 2016).

Enza D'Auria, Diego G. Peroni, Marco Ugo Andrea Sartorio, et al., "The Role of Diet Diversity and Diet Indices on Allergy Outcomes," *Frontiers in Pediatrics* 8 (September 2020): 545, eCollection 2020, https://doi.org/10.3389/fped.2020.00545.

Debra De Silva, Susanne Halken, Chris Singh, et al., "Preventing Food Allergy in Infancy and Childhood: Systematic Review of Randomised Controlled Trials," *Pediatric Allergy and Immunology* 31, no. 7 (October 2020): 813–826, Epub June 18, 2020, https://doi.org/10.1111/pai.13273.

Ing-Mari Dohrn, Lydia Kwak, Pekka Oja, et al., "Replacing Sedentary Time with Physical Activity: A 15-Year Follow-Up of Mortality in a National Cohort," *Clinical Epidemiology* 10 (2018): 179, https://doi.org/10.2147/CLEP.S151613.

Environmental Working Group, "Consumer Guides," https://www.ewg.org/consumer-guides.

Jane Grundy, Sharon Matthews, Belinda Bateman, et al., "Rising Prevalence of Allergy to Peanut in Children: Data from 2 Sequential Cohorts," *Journal of Allergy and Clinical Immunology* 110, no. 5 (November 2002): 784789, https://doi.org/10.1067/mai.2002.128802.

Ruchi S. Gupta, Lucy A. Bilaver, Jacqueline L. Johnson, et al., "Assessment of Pediatrician Awareness and Implementation of the Addendum Guidelines for the Prevention of Peanut Allergy in the United States," *JAMA Network Open* 3, no. 7 (July 2020): e2010511, https://doi.org/10.1001/jamanetworkopen.2020.10511.

Ruchi S. Gupta, Anne Marie Singh, Madeline Walkner, et al., "Hygiene Factors Associated with Childhood Food Allergy and Asthma," *Allergy and Asthma Proceedings* 37, no. 6 (November 2016): e140–e146, https://doi.org/10.2500/aap.2016.37.3988.

Ruchi S. Gupta, Elizabeth E. Springston, Bridget Smith, et al., "Geographic Variability of Childhood Food Allergy in the United States," *Clinical Pediatrics* (Phila) 51, no. 9 (September 2012): 856–861, Epub May 17, 2012, https://doi.org/10.1177/0009922812448526.

Bill Hesselmar, Anna Hicke-Roberts, Anna-Carin Lundell, et al., "Pet-Keeping in Early Life Reduces the Risk of Allergy in a Dose-Dependent Fashion," *PLoS One* 13, no. 12 (December 2018): e0208472, eCollection 2018, https://doi.org/10.1371/journal.pone.0208472.

Bill Hesselmar, Fei Sjöberg, Robert Saalman, et al., "Pacifier Cleaning Practices and Risk of Allergy Development," *Pediatrics* 131, no. 6 (June 2013): e1829–e1837, Epub May 6, 2013, https://doi.org/10.1542/peds.2012-3345.

Galateja Jordakieva, Michael Kundi, Eva Untersmayr, et al., "Country-Wide Medical Records Infer Increased Allergy Risk of Gastric Acid Inhibition," *Nature Communications* 10, no. 1 (July 2019): 3298, https://doi.org/10.1038/s41467-019-10914-6.

J. J. Koplin, S. C. Dharmage, A.-L. Ponsonby, et al., "Environmental and Demographic Risk Factors for Egg Allergy in a Population-Based Study of Infants," *Allergy* 67, no. 11 (November 2012): 1415–1422, Epub September 7, 2012, https://doi.org/10.1111/all.12015.

Edward Mitre, Apryl Susi, Laura E. Kropp, et al., "Association Between Use of Acid-Suppressive Medications and Antibiotics During Infancy and Allergic Diseases in Early Childhood," *JAMA Pediatrics* 172, no. 6 (June 2018): e180315, Epub June 4, 2018, https://doi.org/10.1001/jamapediatrics.2018.0315.

Jennifer N. Morey, Ian A. Boggero, April B. Scott, and Suzanne C. Segerstrom, "Current Directions in Stress and Human Immune Function," *Current Opinion in Psychology* 5 (October 2015): 13–17, https://doi.org/10.1016/j.copsyc.2015.03.007.

Christina L. Nance, Roman Deniskin, Veronica C. Diaz, et al., "The Role of the Microbiome in Food Allergy: A Review," *Children* (Basel) 7, no. 6 (May 2020): 50, https://doi.org/10.3390/children7060050.

National Academies of Sciences, Engineering, and Medicine; Health and Medicine Division; Food and Nutrition Board; Committee on Food Allergies: Global Burden, Causes, Treatment, Prevention, and Public Policy, "Finding a Path to Safety in Food Allergy: Assessment of the Global Burden, Causes, Prevention, Management, and Public Policy," eds. M. P. Oria and V. A. Stallings (Washington, DC: National Academies Press, November 30, 2016), PMID: 28609025.

Nature.com, "Scientists Swab C-Section-Babies with Mothers' Microbes," https://www.nature.com/news/scientists-swab-c-section-babies-with-mothers-microbes-1.19275.

David C. Nieman and Laurel M. Wentz, "The Compelling Link Between Physical Activity and the Body's Defense System," *Journal of Sport and Health Science* 8, no. 3 (May 2019): 201–217, Epub November 16, 2018, https://doi.org/10.1016/j.jshs.2018.09.009.

Berthe C. Oosterloo, Arine M. Vlieger, and Ruurd M. van Elburg, "Antibiotics and Acid-Suppressing Medications in Early Life and Allergic Disorders," *JAMA Pediatrics* 172, no. 10 (October 2018): 988–989, https://doi.org/10.1001/jamapediatrics.2018.2520.

Michael R. Perkin, Kirsty Logan, Tom Marrs, et al., "Enquiring About Tolerance (EAT) Study: Feasibility of an Early Allergenic Food Introduction Regimen," *Journal of Allergy and Clinical Immunology* 137, no. 5 (May 2016): 1477–1486.e8, Epub February 17, 2016, https://doi.org/10.1016/j.jaci.2015.12.1322.

Caroline Roduit, Remo Frei, Martin Depner, et al., "Increased Food Diversity in the First Year of Life Is Inversely Associated with Allergic Diseases," *Journal of Allergy and Clinical Immunology* 133, no. 4 (April 2014): 1056–1064, Epub February 6, 2014, https://doi.org/10.1016/j.jaci.2013.12.1044.

Menachem Rottem, World Allergy Organization, "Vaccination and the Risk of Atopy and Asthma," June 2011; updated September 2016, https://www.worldallergy.org/education-and-programs/education/allergic-disease-resource-center/professionals/vaccination-and-the-risk-of-atopy-and-asthma.

Waheeda Samady, Emily Campbell, Ozge Nur Aktas, et al., "Recommendations on Complementary Food Introduction Among Pediatric Practitioners," *JAMA Network Open* 3, no. 8 (August 2020): e2013070, https://doi.org/10.1001/jamanetworkopen.2020.13070.

A. Schroeder, R. Kumar, J. A. Pongracic, et al., "Food Allergy Is Associated with an Increased Risk of Asthma," *Clinical and Experimental Allergy* 39, no. 2 (February 2009): 261–270, https://doi.org/10.1111/j.1365-2222.2008.03160.x.

Megan Scudellari, "News Feature: Cleaning Up the Hygiene Hypothesis," *Proc Natl Acad Sci USA* 114, no. 7 (February 2017): 1433–1436, https://doi.org/10.1073/pnas.1700688114.

Elinor Simons, Robert Balshaw, Diana L. Lefebvre, et al., "Timing of Introduction, Sensitization, and Allergy to Highly Allergenic Foods at Age 3 Years in a General-Population Canadian Cohort," *Journal of Allergy and Clinical Immunology in Practice* 8, no. 1 (January 2020): 166–175.e10, Epub October 31, 2019, https://doi.org/10.1016/j.jaip.2019.09.039.

Sleepfoundation.org.

Jackie Swartz, Bernice Aronsson, Frank Lindblad, et al., "Vaccination and Allergic Sensitization in Early Childhood—The ALADDIN Birth Cohort," *EClinicalMedicine* (November 2018): 92–98, eCollection October–November 2018, https://doi.org/10.1016/j.eclinm.2018.10.005.

Maxwell M. Tran, Diana L. Lefebvre, Christoffer Dharma, et al., "Predicting the Atopic March: Results from the Canadian Healthy Infant Longitudinal Development Study," *Journal of Allergy and Clinical Immunology* 141, no. 2 (February 2018): 601–607.e8, Epub November 15, 2017, https://doi.org/10.1016/j.jaci.2017.08.024.

D. Venkataraman, M. Erlewyn-Lajeunesse, R. J. Kurukulaaratchy, et al., "Prevalence and Longitudinal Trends of Food Allergy During Childhood and Adolescence: Results of the Isle of Wight Birth Cohort Study," *Clinical and Experimental Allergy* 48, no. 4 (April 2018): 394–402, Epub February 8, 2018, https://doi.org/10.1111/cea.13088.

Carina Venter, Carlo Agostoni, S. Hasan Arshad, et al., "Dietary Factors During Pregnancy and Atopic Outcomes in Childhood: A Systematic Review from the European Academy of Allergy and Clinical Immunology," *Pediatric Allergy and Immunology* 31, no. 8 (November 2020): 889–912, Epub August 6, 2020, https://doi.org/10.1111/pai.13303.

Carina Venter, Kate Maslin, John W. Holloway, et al., "Different Measures of Diet Diversity During Infancy and the Association with Childhood Food Allergy in a UK Birth Cohort Study," *Journal of Allergy and Clinical Immunology in Practice* 8, no. 6 (June 2020): 2017–2026, Epub January 28, 2020, https://doi.org/10.1016/j.jaip.2020.01.029.

Carina Venter, Matthew Greenhawt, Rosan W. Meyer, et al., "EAACI Position Paper on Diet Diversity in Pregnancy, Infancy and Childhood: Novel Concepts and Implications for Studies in Allergy and Asthma," *Allergy* 75, no. 3 (March 2020): 497–523, https://doi.org/10.1111/all.14051.

Matthew Walker, *Why We Sleep: Unlocking the Power of Sleep and Dreams* (New York: Scribner, 2017).

Gabriela Wlasiuk and Donata Vercelli, "The Farm Effect, or: When, What and How a Farming Environment Protects from Asthma and Allergic Disease," *Current Opinion in Allergy and Clinical Immunology* 12, no. 5 (October 2012): 461–466, https://doi.org/10.1097/ACI.0b013e328357a3bc.

Justin M. Zaslavsky, Waheeda Samady, Jialing Jiang, et al., "Family History of Atopy in Food Allergy Development," *Journal of Allergy and Clinical Immunology* 143, no. 2 (February 2019): suppl. AB83.

CHAPTER 9: Thrive in Your Daily World:
Cracking the Label Codes and Building Confidence to Live Fearlessly

Allergic Living, "Top Allergens: Places Where They Hide," https://www.allergicliving.com/2010/09/01/hidden-allergens/.

Matthew Greenhawt, Fiona MacGillivray, Geraldine Batty, et al., "International Study of Risk-Mitigating Factors and In-Flight Allergic Reactions to

Peanut and Tree Nut," *Journal of Allergy and Clinical Immunology in Practice* 1, no. 2 (March 2013): 186–194, Epub February 26, 2013, https://doi.org/10.1016/j.jaip.2013.01.002.

Heather MacKenzie, Jane Grundy, Gillian Glasbey, et al., "Information and Support from Dietary Consultation for Mothers of Children with Food Allergies," *Annals of Allergy, Asthma & Immunology* 114, no. 1 (January 2015): 23–29, Epub October 25, 2014, https://doi.org/10.1016/j.anai.2014.10.001.

Please see comprehensive list of studies on my website at https://www.feinberg.northwestern.edu/faculty-profiles/az/profile.html?xid=17229#publications.

CHAPTER 10: Act Locally, Think Globally:
What We Can Do as a Society to Turn This Epidemic Around

Centers for Disease Control and Prevention, "Voluntary Guidelines for Managing Food Allergies in Schools and Early Care and Education Programs," https://www.cdc.gov/healthyschools/foodallergies/pdf/Food_Allergy_Guidelines_FAQs.pdf.

Global News Wire, "Allergy Treatment Market to Garner $40.36 Billion by 2026," February 13, 2020, https://www.globenewswire.com/news-release/2020/02/13/1984673/0/en/Allergy-Treatment-Market-to-Garner-40-36-Billion-by-2026.html.

Abrahm Lustgarten, "How Climate Change Is Contributing to Skyrocketing Rates of Infectious Disease," ProPublica.org, https://www.propublica.org/article/climate-infectious-diseases.

INDEX